FULL MOUTH
DENTAL IMPLANTS
FOR THE
CURIOUS PATIENT

Sal
Thanks for all your help
& support. Couldn't do
this without you

DR ISAAC QURESHI

All works presented are opinions of Dr Isaac Qureshi, and are not to be presented as sole options or should be taken as scientific evidence or considered as such. Though almost all of the opinions are backed by scientific data.

Copyright © 2024 by Isaac Qureshi

All Rights reserved. No part of this book may be reproduced or used in any manner without the written permission of the copyright owner except for the use of quotations in book review.

First Edition March 2024

ISBN 979-8-218-37992-6

CONTENTS

CHAPTER 01
    INTRODUCTION   1

CHAPTER 02
    WHAT ARE TEETH?   7

CHAPTER 03
    WHY DOES MY MOUTH HURT?   14

CHAPTER 04
    MODERN RESTORATIVE DENTISTRY   22

CHAPTER 05
    ALL ON X: EVERYTHING BEFORE SURGERY   31

CHAPTER 06
    SURGERY DAY   43

CHAPTER 07
    AFTER SURGERY AND BEYOND   56

CONCLUSIONS: 66

ABOUT THE AUTHOR   67

CHAPTER 01

INTRODUCTION

This book is designed for the curious patient eager to explore options for rejuvenating or replacing their teeth. Teeth can deteriorate for a variety of reasons, and we will explore these causes throughout our discussion. If you find yourself considering the removal of all your teeth in favor of dental implants, there are several approaches you can take. The primary focus of this book is the All-on-X procedure, also known as all-on-4, hybrid dentures, or full mouth fixed implants.

This book aims to equip you with a thorough understanding of what to expect, presenting alternatives and equipping you with the knowledge needed to make an informed decision about your treatment.

It is important to note that this book is not intended as a guide for dentists on how to perform these procedures, nor does it claim to answer every possible question. However, it offers sufficient information to help you identify the ideal treatment for your needs, making you an informed patient ready to embark on your dental restoration journey.

Introduction

All on X Overview

An All-on-X procedure essentially utilizes the minimum number of implants required to fully restore your chewing capability. I personally recommend the placement of six implants in the upper jaw and five implants in the lower jaw. This is because bone density in the upper jaw is typically lower than that in the lower jaw.

Opting for a treatment like this not only results in aesthetically pleasing teeth but also significantly enhances the interaction between the jaw muscles and the teeth. This leads to a more comfortable and natural feeling during use, closely mimicking the function of natural teeth and optimizing oral health.

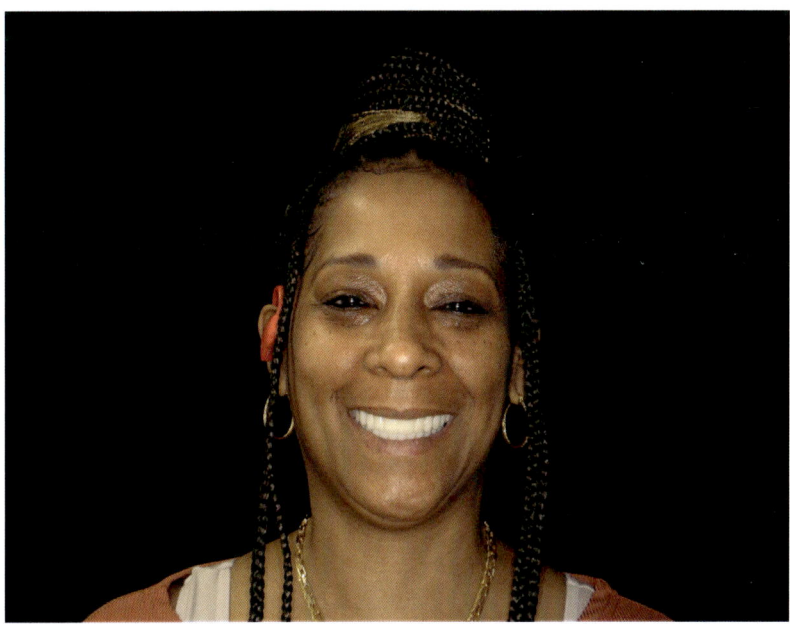

Where should I get the surgery done?

Numerous clinics both within and outside the United States offer All-on-X dental implants. Many individuals are tempted by the prospect of undergoing these procedures abroad, attracted by the lower costs. However, it's important to consider that while initial expenses might be reduced, the cost of addressing any complications that arise later could significantly increase.

When choosing a location for your dental work, it is essential to weigh several factors carefully: the quality of the work, the cost, and the expertise of the dental team. Avoid making a decision based solely on convenience or the first option you come across. Instead, ensure you feel comfortable and confident with your choice.

To make an informed decision, it's advisable to review a comprehensive portfolio of before and after photos, inquire about the technology utilized by the clinic, and consider patient testimonials and reviews.

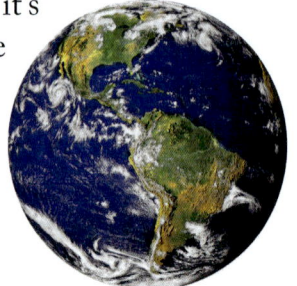

Introduction | 4

How many implants should I have?

Finding a straightforward answer in the context of dental implants, particularly the number required for optimal results, is challenging. While four implants might suffice for some patients, it's essential to recognize that no two surgeries are identical. Every individual's needs vary, making each mouth restoration unique.

Therefore, the decision regarding the number of implants should be entrusted to a team of skilled and experienced professionals. Their expertise ensures that the treatment plan is tailored to meet the specific requirements of each patient, ensuring the best possible outcome.

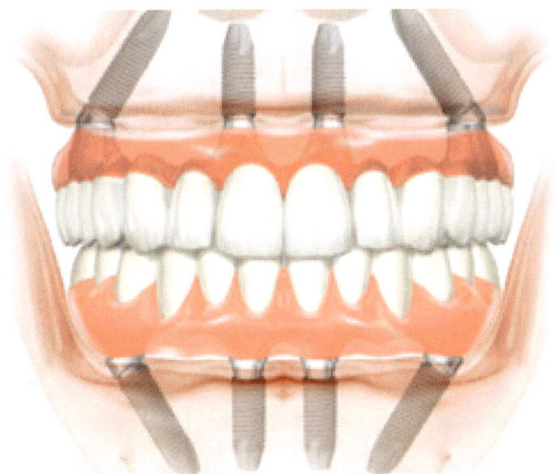

Digital vs analog

When choosing a dental office for your procedure, it's crucial to inquire about the process for fitting the initial temporary teeth post-surgery, specifically whether they employ digital or analog methods. We advocate for digital techniques as the preferred approach moving forward, although we will also discuss analog methods later in the book.

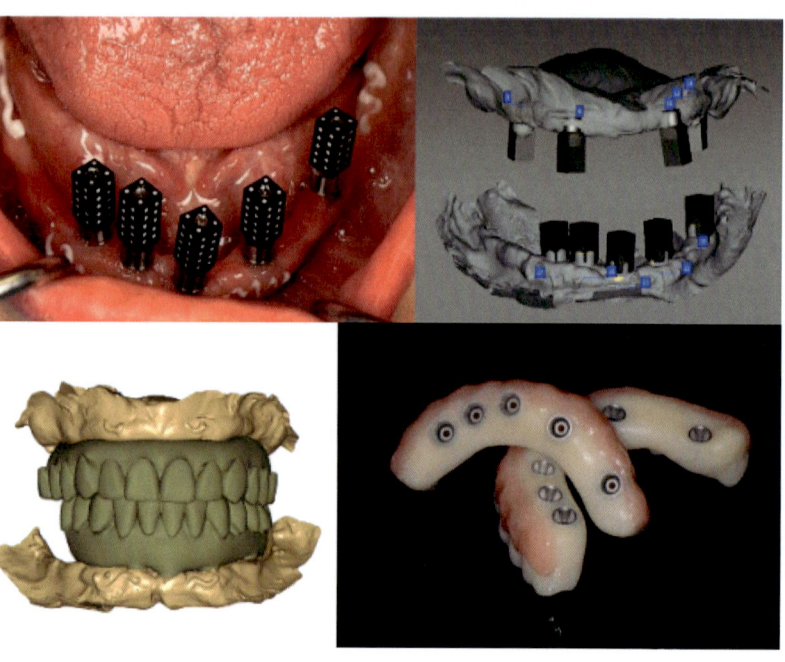

Introduction

Zirconia teeth vs Acrylic fused to metal

Zirconia represents a relatively new advancement in dental materials. To my patients, I often describe it as a metal with the aesthetic appeal of white porcelain, combining the durability of metal with the beauty of porcelain. This contrasts with the traditional option of a titanium bar overlaid with plastic acrylic teeth. Despite some issues associated with Zirconia, which I will detail later, I recommend it because the potential complications are generally more manageable compared to those associated with traditional acrylic fused to metal frameworks.

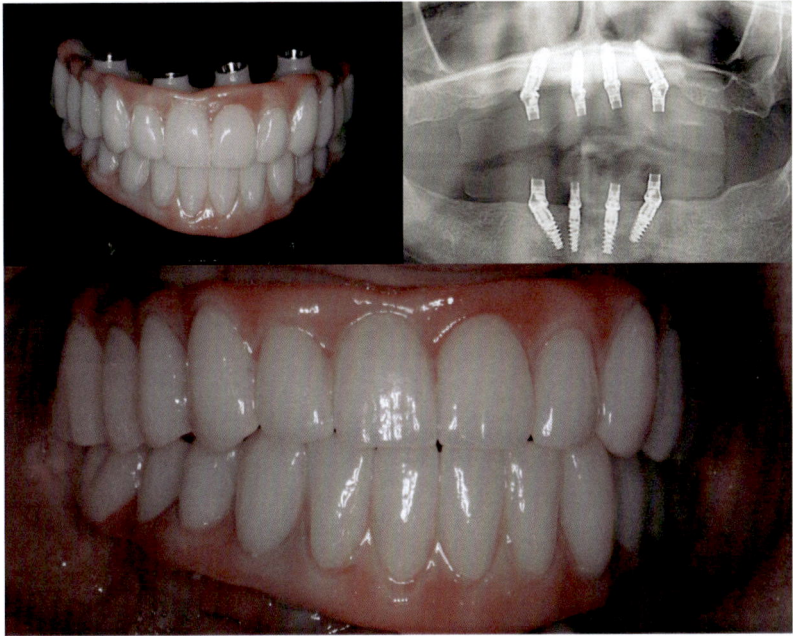

CHAPTER 02

WHAT ARE TEETH?

What is the purpose of teeth?

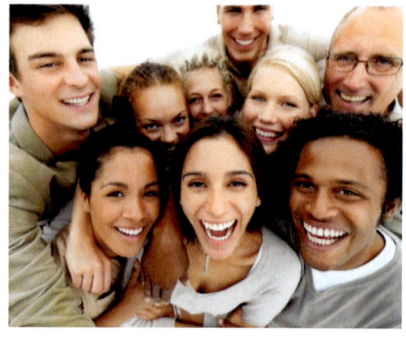

Teeth are often the most overlooked human organ, yet their value becomes profoundly appreciated during times of distress. In my view, the primary function of teeth is to facilitate proper digestion and nutrition. Consuming a balanced diet, aided by effective chewing, is crucial for overall health and well-being.

Beyond their functional role, teeth play a significant part in emotional expression, showcasing feelings of happiness, joy, and even sadness. Damage to teeth can not only impair physical health but also lead to psychological discomfort. Many individuals with dental issues may feel self-conscious or embarrassed. This underscores the importance of dental health not just for physical well-being but for emotional and psychological health as well.

What Are Teeth?

People are born with 32 teeth

Teeth are composed of several types, each serving a unique function. The front part of the mouth contains six teeth known as incisors and canines—four incisors for cutting and two canines for tearing food. Adjacent to the canines are the premolars (bicuspids), typically two on each side, which crush and tear food. Beyond the premolars, there are the molars, including three on each side of both the upper and lower jaws, which make up the back teeth.

Teeth are organized into two arches: the upper arch and the lower arch. Aesthetically, the front six teeth, which span from canine to canine, are considered the most important due to their visibility and impact on one's smile. Functionally, the molars play a crucial role in digestion by performing the bulk of chewing.

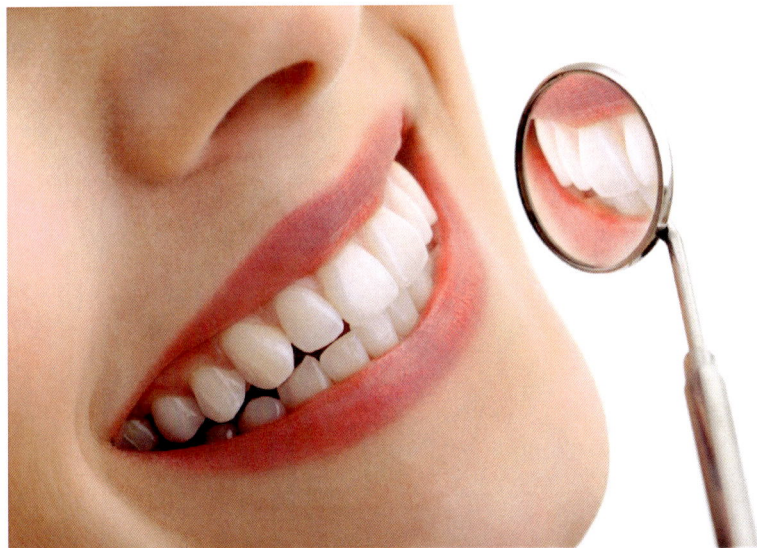

Chewing is more than just the teeth

A frequently overlooked aspect of the chewing pro-cess involves not only the teeth but also the skull that houses them, the muscles that facilitate chewing and smiling, and the temporo-mandibular joint (TMJ) that orchestrates the movement of this system. While it's not necessary to delve into the intricacies of every muscle involved, awareness of their existence and role is essential. Reconstructing these complex systems goes beyond mere tooth replacement; it requires a deep appreciation for the intricate anatomy and functions that most people are naturally equipped with. Understanding this complexity is crucial in appreciating the full scope of dental and facial anatomy.

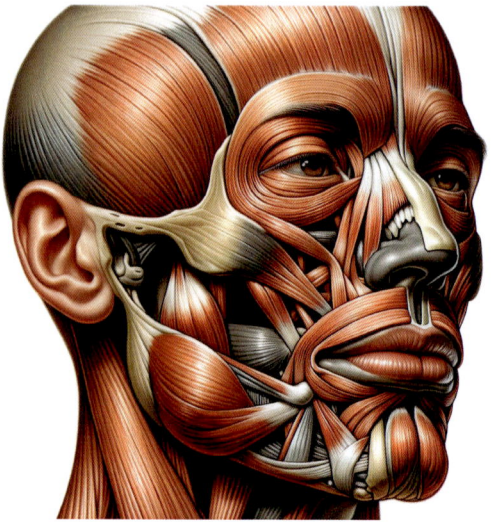

What Are Teeth? | 10

Appreciate the Skull

While the upper and lower sets of teeth function independently, they are part of a sophisticated system that includes the muscles, the skull, and the teeth themselves, all intricately working together to enable efficient chewing. The lower jaw (mandible) and the rest of the skull, facilitating movement and serving as a protective mechanism. It is not merely a connector but also ensures that movements of the jaw are smooth and coordinated, enabling activities such as chewing, speaking, and yawning.

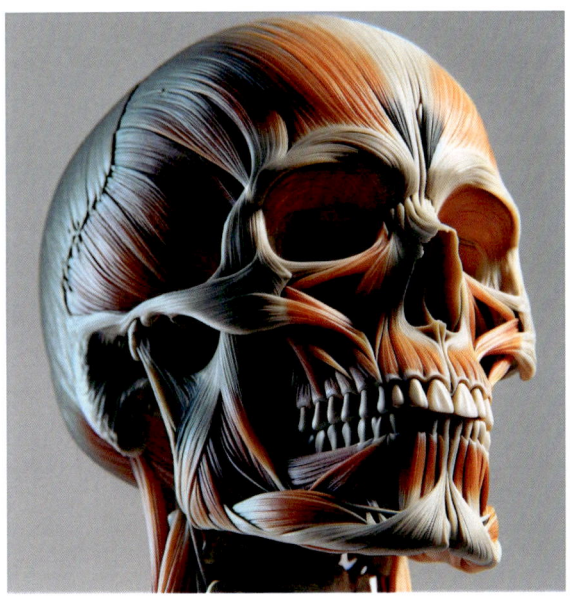

11 What Are Teeth?

Anatomical considerations:

In surgical procedures, we have to account for several anatomical features to minimize complications. These include the nerves and blood vessels, marked by an orange line for identification, which are vital for sensory and nourishment. Damage to these structures can result in numbness, pain, or bleeding. The sinus cavities, highlighted in purple, are carefully considered due to their proximity to upper teeth extractions or implants. Breaching these cavities can lead to sinusitis. Furthermore, the nasal area, delineated with a yellow highlight, demands attention to avoid impairing nasal structure or function, which could affect breathing or cause infections.

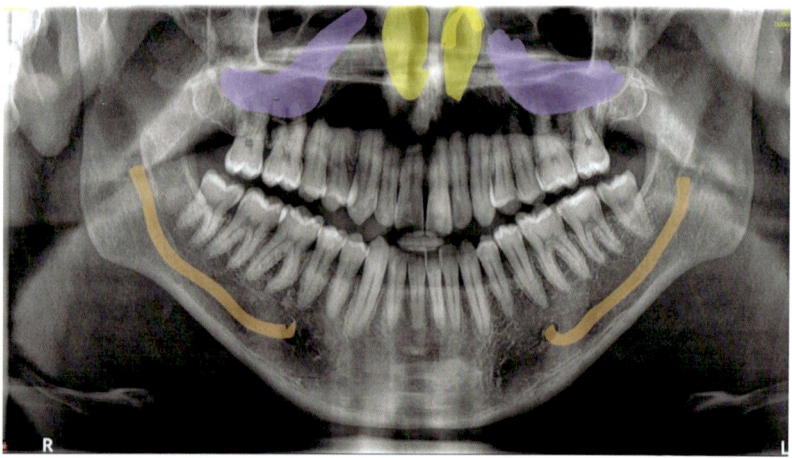

What Are Teeth? | 12

Problems with Teeth- Cavities:

Tooth cavities, also known as dental caries, represent one of the most prevalent and significant health issues globally. These cavities arise from the acidic by-products produced by bacteria in the mouth, which consume the sugars we ingest. This process initiates the erosion and decay of tooth enamel, leading to the formation of cavities. When detected early, cavities are typically manageable through fillings, a process that restores the tooth's integrity and prevents further damage. However, if left unchecked, cavities can expand, necessitating more invasive treatments such as root canals or crowns. In severe cases, extensive decay may lead to tooth loss.

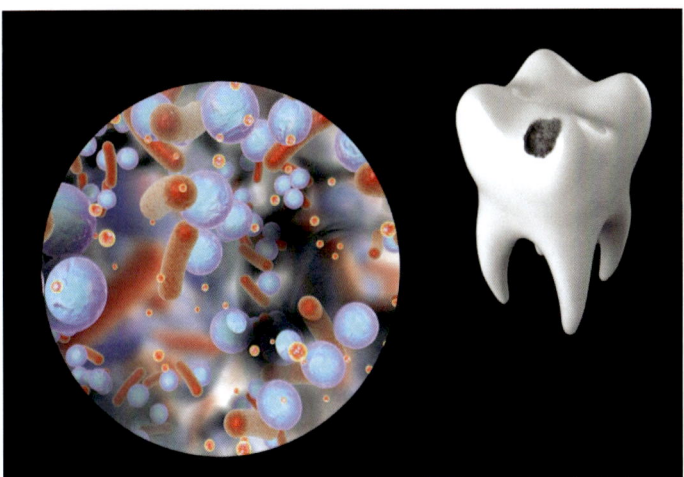

Problems with Teeth- Gum Disease:

Gum disease, also known as periodontal disease, is a significant health concern characterized by inflammation of the gums, which can lead to bone loss and, if untreated, eventual tooth loss. This condition is primarily caused by specific bacteria that infect the gums, often exacerbated by inadequate oral hygiene. However, genetics can also play a role in an individual's susceptibility to periodontal disease. One of the most concerning aspects of gum disease is its established link to heart disease, highlighting the critical importance of maintaining optimal oral health not only for the preservation of overall health.

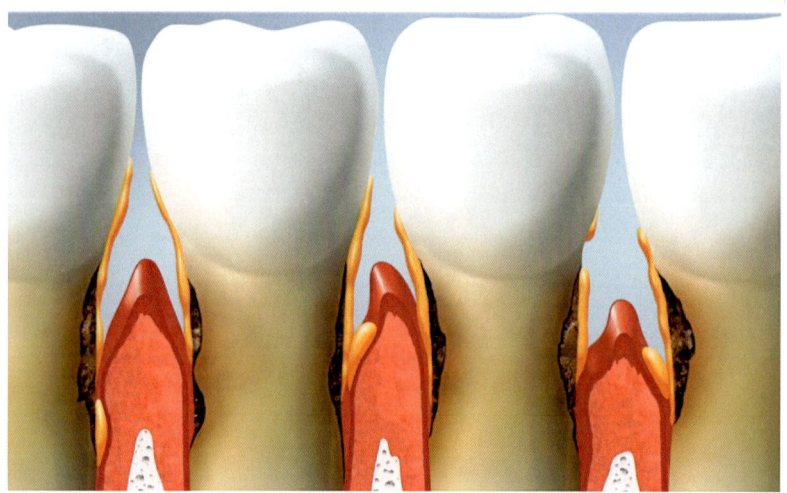

CHAPTER 03

WHY DOES MY MOUTH HURT?

Cavities and pain:

One prevalent source of tooth pain is nerve discomfort, which typically occurs when a cavity enlarges and approaches the nerves located at the tooth's core. This proximity to the nerves, which are directly connected to the nervous system and ultimately the brain, is primarily responsible for the sensation of tooth pain. As the decay progresses closer to these sensitive areas, it can trigger significant discomfort, underscoring the importance of addressing cavities early to prevent the onset of nerve pain.

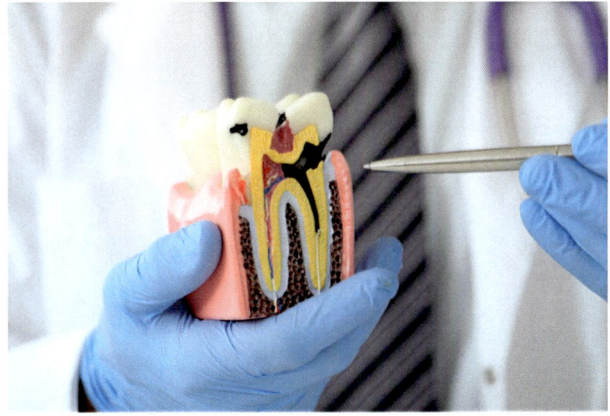

Abscesses and pain:

Over time, if left untreated, the nerve subjected to decay and damage can eventually die. This dead tissue then begins to form an abscess beneath the tooth, marking the onset of even more severe pain. If this condition remains unaddressed, the infection can spread to other tissues within the mouth and has the potential to travel to the brain, posing a fatal risk. This progression highlights the critical importance of timely dental intervention to prevent the escalation from severe discomfort to life-threatening complications.

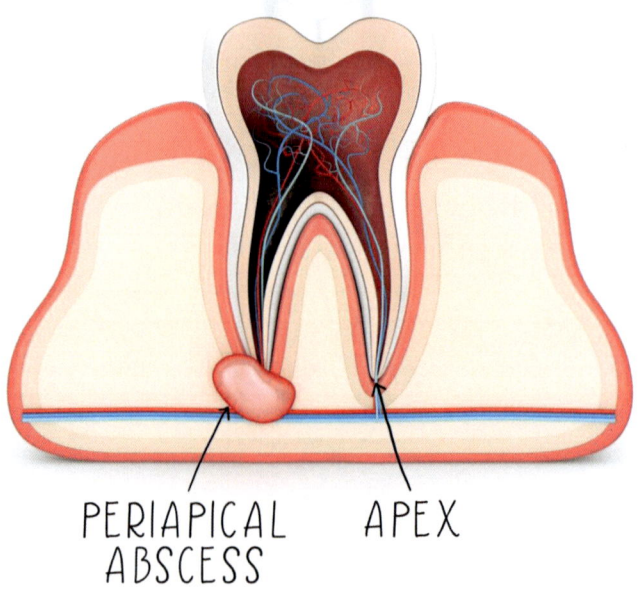

PERIAPICAL ABSCESS   APEX

Why Does My Mouth Hurt? 16

Gum disease and pain:

As gum disease progresses, it creates more opportunities for bacteria to flourish, exacerbating the swelling and inflammation. In its advanced stages, gum disease can even lead to the formation of abscesses, which are pockets of infection that pose serious health risks. In response to these infections, the body's defense mechanisms may activate, sometimes resulting in tooth loss as a means to eliminate the source of infection. This highlights the importance of early detection and treatment of gum disease to prevent its progression to more severe outcomes.

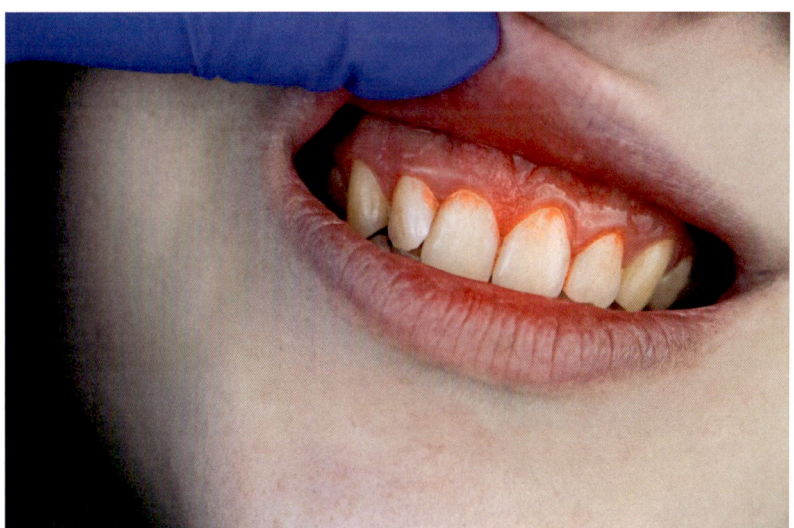

Swelling and pain:

We have explored the primary causes of swelling associated with dental conditions, highlighting how inflammation can progressively worsen. While antibiotics serve as a temporary measure to alleviate symptoms, their effectiveness can be delayed in cases of severe infections. Personally, witnessing uncontrolled infections in the dental office is among the most daunting experiences. Such infections, if not promptly and effectively managed, can lead to extended stays in the Intensive Care Unit (ICU), spanning months, as the body struggles to combat the infection. This scenario underscores the critical need for early intervention and comprehensive care to prevent infections from reaching a point where they pose a significant threat to health.

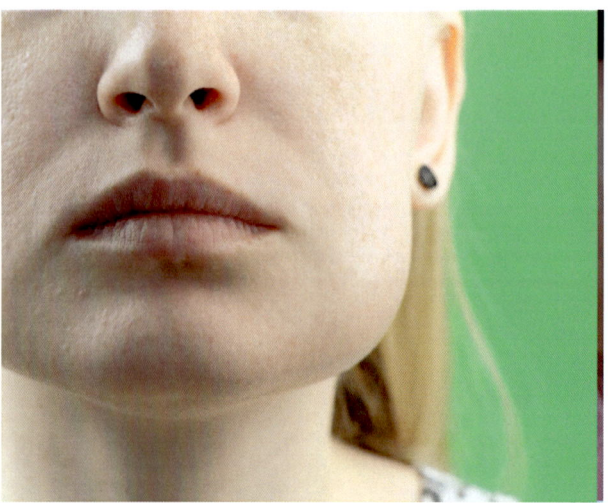

Muscle and Joint pain:

Another prevalent source of facial discomfort stems from abnormalities in the TMJ joint or the muscles that support it. Various factors can contribute to this condition, with the most frequent being a misalignment between the teeth and the skull. Ideally, the movements of the skull and the alignment of the teeth should complement each other seamlessly. However, discrepancies between these two can lead to significant discomfort, often manifesting as pain near the ears or on the sides of the head, particularly noticeable upon waking. This issue can also be a contributing factor to many cases of headaches, including those often misdiagnosed as migraines, highlighting the importance of considering dental interactions in the differential diagnosis of head pain.

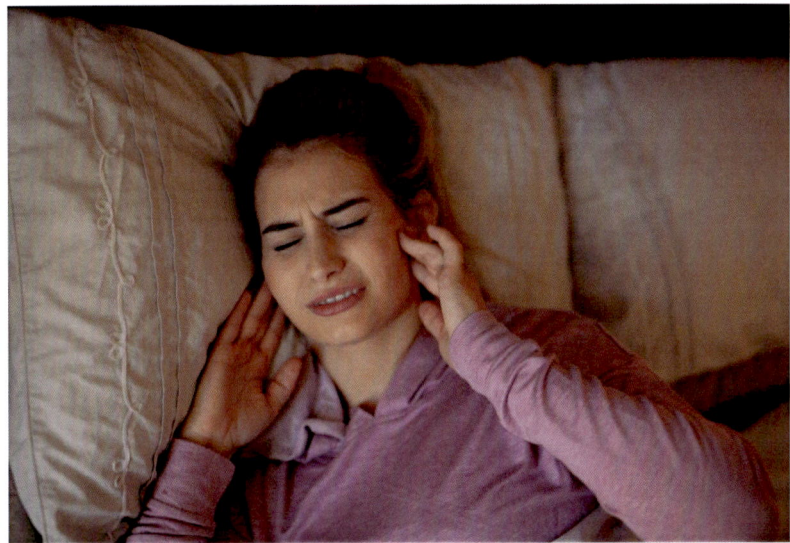

Nerve Pain: Nerve Injury

There are several types of nerve pain associated with dental health. A frequent cause of such pain is nerve damage incurred during dental procedures. This damage can occur in various ways, including accidental injury, severance, or stretching of nerves during treatment. Additionally, accidents or other forms of trauma can directly harm dental nerves.

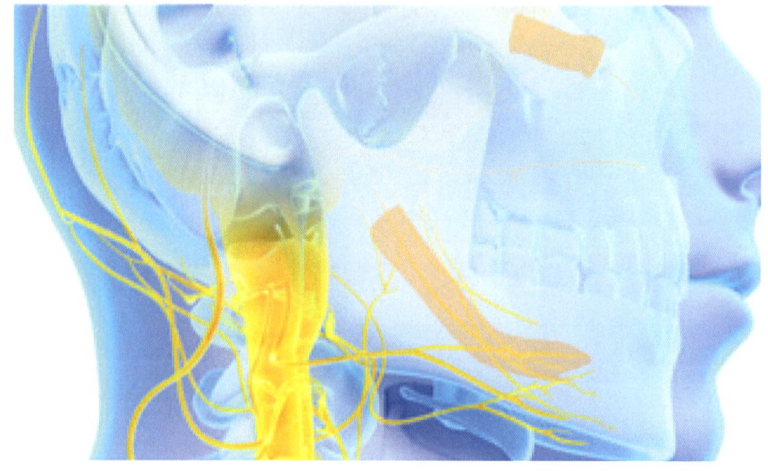

Nerve Pain: Neurological:

One of the most cha-llenging types of pain to diagnose and treat is referred nerve pain. This complexity arises because many dental issues are misattributed to it, stemming from the brain's capacity to mislead the body into perceiving pain where it may not directly exist. The brain, with its incredible complexity and still not fully understood mechanisms, can create scenarios where both patients and dentists find themselves perplexed by the symptoms presented.

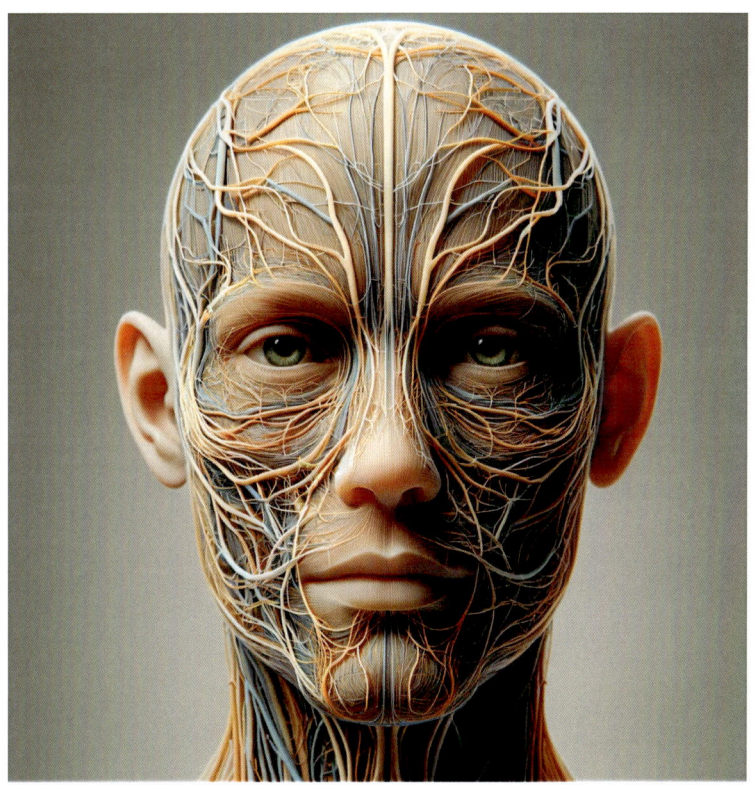

Pain: Accident or Trauma

Occasionally, individuals who have diligently maintained their oral health may still suffer dental damage due to accidents or trauma. Treating patients affected by these circumstances presents unique challenges, especially when the teeth appeared to be in excellent condition prior to the injury and may still seem visually unaffected afterward. However, it's important to recognize that symptoms resulting from trauma may not manifest immediately; instead, they can take months or even years to develop, necessitating a vigilant and proactive approach to dental care in the aftermath of such incidents.

CHAPTER 04

MODERN RESTORATIVE DENTISTRY

Terminal Dentition:

Delving into the myriad ways dentists can repair teeth could fill volumes, so we'll set aside those details for the moment. Instead, our focus shifts to the concept of full teeth replacement. Terminal dentition occurs when the dentist and patient collaboratively determine that the teeth are beyond salvage, a decision influenced by a variety of factors previously discussed. At this juncture, critical choices must be made regarding the best path forward for restoring oral health and functionality. This part of our discussion will concentrate on the options available for those facing the prospect of replacing all their teeth, exploring the most effective strategies to ensure a return to both aesthetic appeal and dental function.

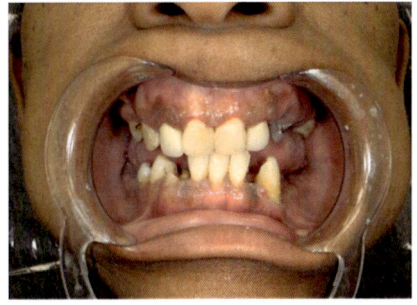

Partial Dentures

While acknowledging the historical significance of partial dentures in dental treatment, it's important to recognize their limitations. A partial denture, a removable appliance tailored to an individual's mouth, often inadvertently exerts additional pressure on the abutment teeth — those to which the denture is attached. Ideally, their use should be constrained by financial or health considerations and viewed as a temporary solution. Prolonged reliance on partial dentures can lead to the need for frequent replacements and might culminate in the eventual transition to complete dentures. Thus, when exploring dental restoration options, it's advisable to consider alternatives that minimize undue stress on remaining natural teeth and offer a more sustainable solution for the long term.

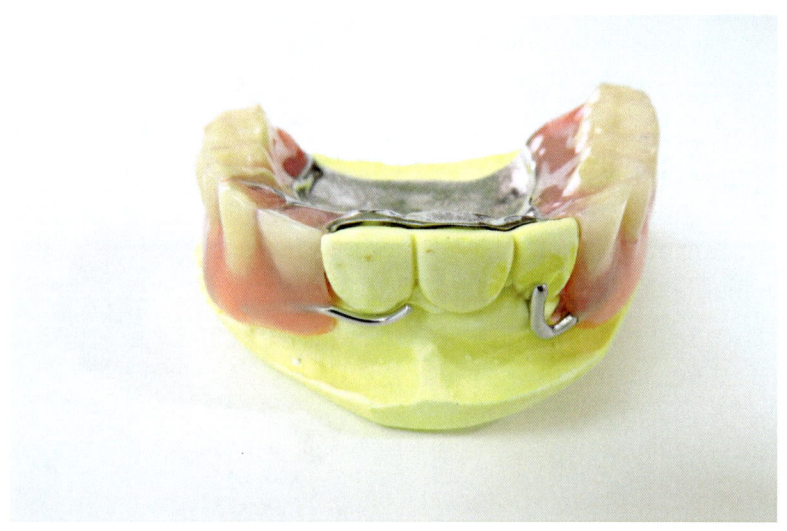

Modern Restorative Dentistry | 24

Complete Dentures

Complete dentures, with a history tracing back to the 7th century, have been a staple in dental prosthetics for centuries. Despite the advent of modern materials, the fundamental design of plastic dentures has remained relatively unchanged over the past 50 to 75 years. These dentures rest on the soft tissue of the mouth, with lower dentures presenting particular challenges in terms of stability and often necessitating the use of glues. Notably, the force exerted during chewing with natural teeth can reach 200-250 pounds, whereas with dentures, this force significantly reduces to about 40-60 pounds. This reduction means that the efficiency of chewing with dentures drops to nearly 20% of that with natural teeth.

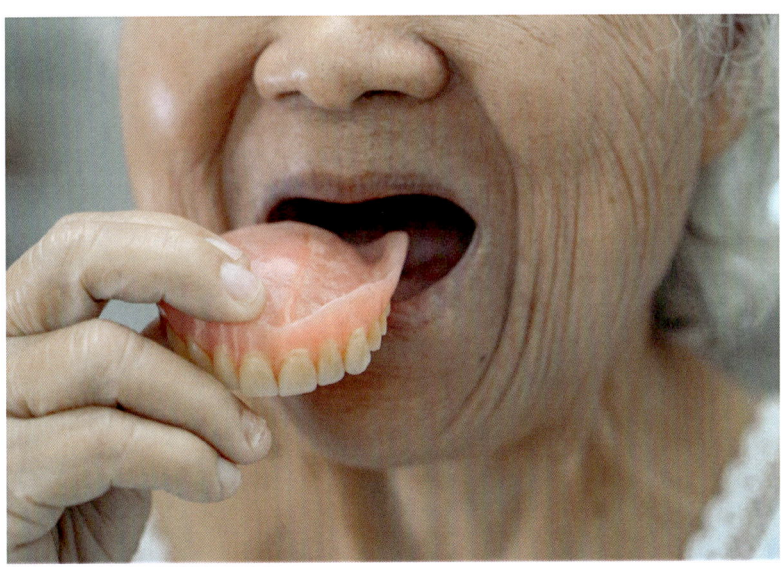

What is a Dental Implant?

Before delving into the transformative potential of dental implants, let's clarify what they entail. A traditional dental implant consists of a sterilized screw, crafted from titanium or, in more recent developments, zirconia. This screw is precisely inserted into the jawbone, ensuring it avoids critical anatomical structures. Following placement, the body naturally integrates the implant, with bone growth occurring within the screw's threads, securely anchoring it to the jaw. This biological fusion not only stabilizes the implant but also forms an anchor that boasts a 97% success rate.

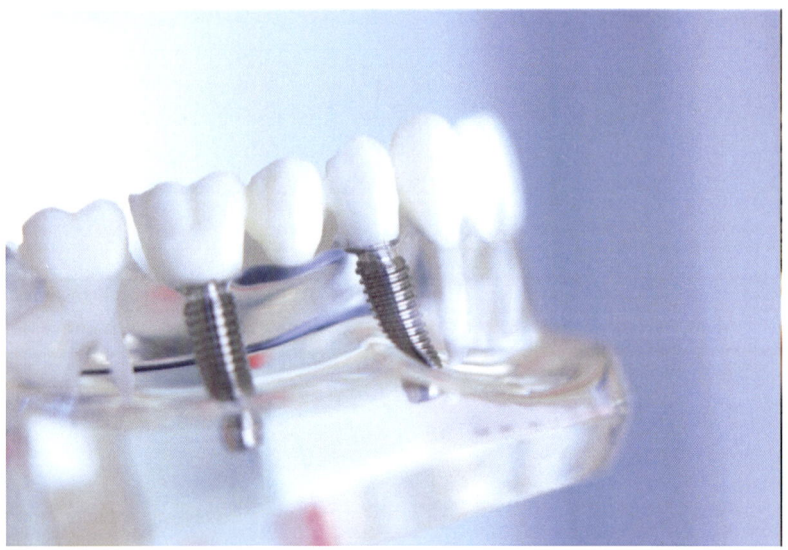

Modern Restorative Dentistry

What can you do with Dental Implants?

Dental implant treatments are broadly categorized into two primary strategies: augmenting or emulating your existing dentition, or serving as a complete replacement.

For localized solutions, a single implant can be utilized to replace an individual tooth or to anchor a dental bridge, effectively addressing specific gaps in your smile. In an ideal scenario, it's conceivable to replace each missing tooth with its own implant, providing a solution that closely mirrors natural dental architecture. The primary constraint of this approach is its cost. A full-mouth restoration, where every tooth is replaced with an individual implant, can be prohibitively expensive, with estimates nearing $100,000 USD.

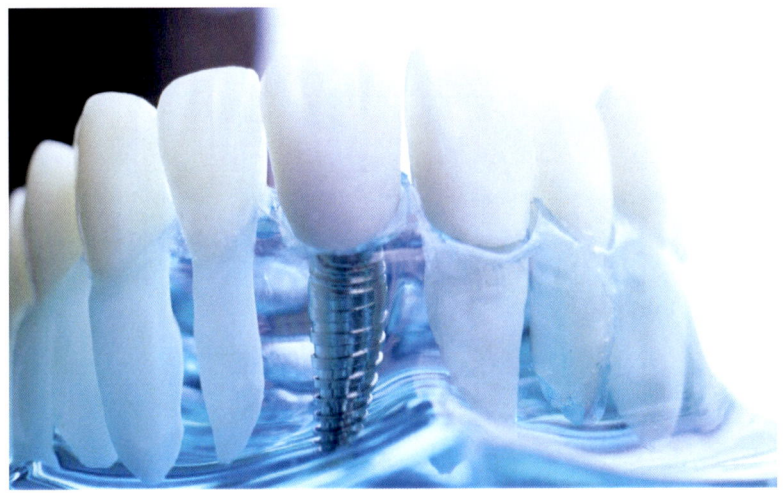

Full mouth Implants: Overdentures

In my view, overdentures represent the most cost-effective approach to replacing all your teeth while providing adequate chewing.. This method typically involves the use of either two implants (for the lower jaw) or at least four implants to securely anchor traditional dentures. While this technique does have its limitations, it successfully replicates approximately 50-60% of natural chewing power, which for many patients, might be the most viable option available.

However, it's important to note that overdentures require removal every night, and are bulkier than their fixed counterparts.

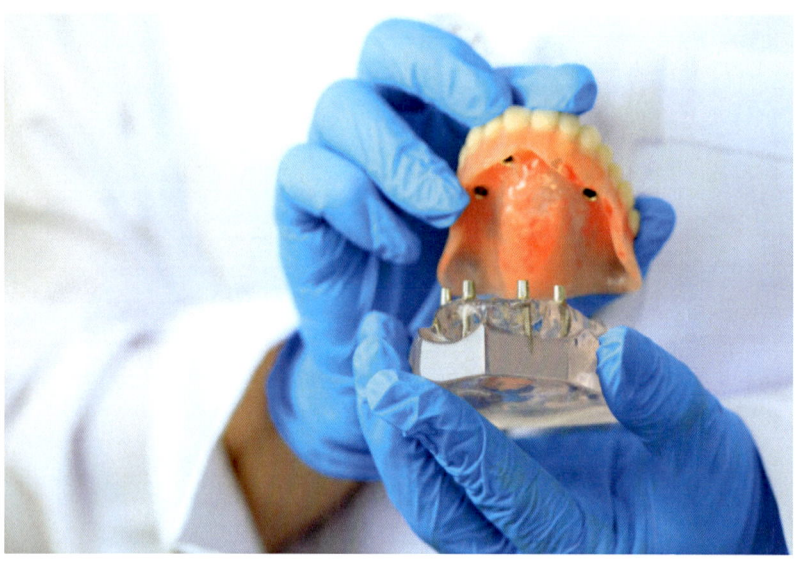

Modern Restorative Dentistry | 28

Full mouth implants: Overdentures cont.

Another significant advantage of overdentures is the ability to clean them daily. Regular maintenance is essential, including the replacement of the plastic inserts (the blue part depicted in illustrations) that secure them in place, as well as ensuring the area around the implants is free from bacteria. Ensuring these components are properly designed and maintained can significantly enhance the longevity and comfort of your overdentures.

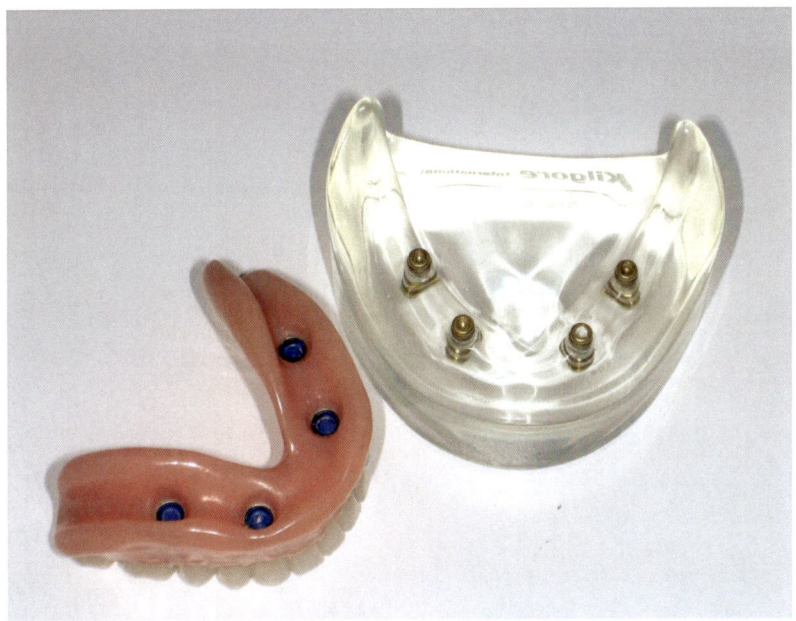

Full mouth implants: Individuals

Placing individual implants represents an optimal solution for replacing teeth, closely replicating the original strength and functionality of your natural dentition. As previously mentioned, this approach does come with a higher cost. However, for those who have the financial means, it is arguably the best method available. Opting for individual implants not only ensures a restoration that feels and functions like natural teeth but also offers long-term benefits in terms of oral health and overall quality of life.

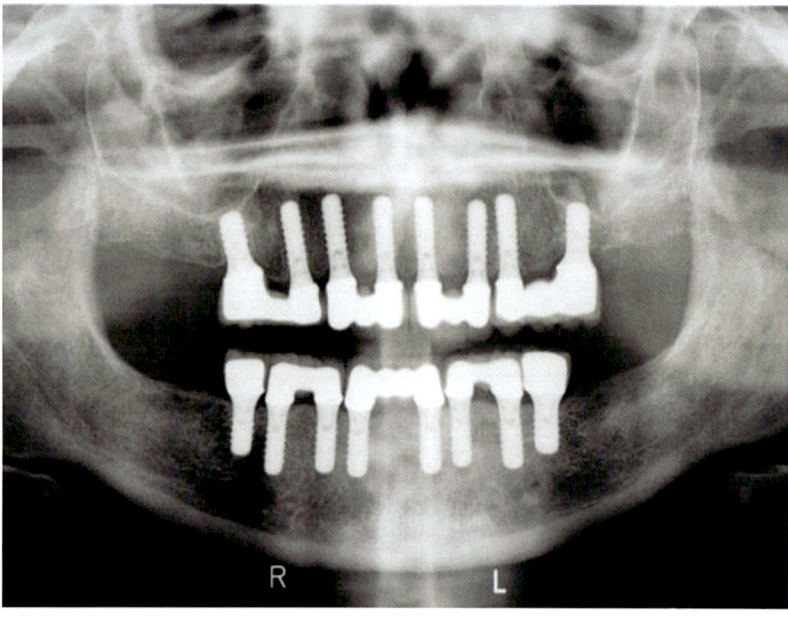

Modern Restorative Dentistry | 30

Full mouth Implants: All on X

The discussion thus far has been building up to this pivotal topic: the All-on-X (typically involving 4 to 6 implants), also known as Hybrid Dentures or simply "Dental Implants." This innovative approach represents a significant advancement in dental restoration techniques. Now, we will delve into a comprehensive exploration of this option, providing detailed insights into its methodology, benefits, and potential impact on those seeking a transformative solution to extensive dental loss.

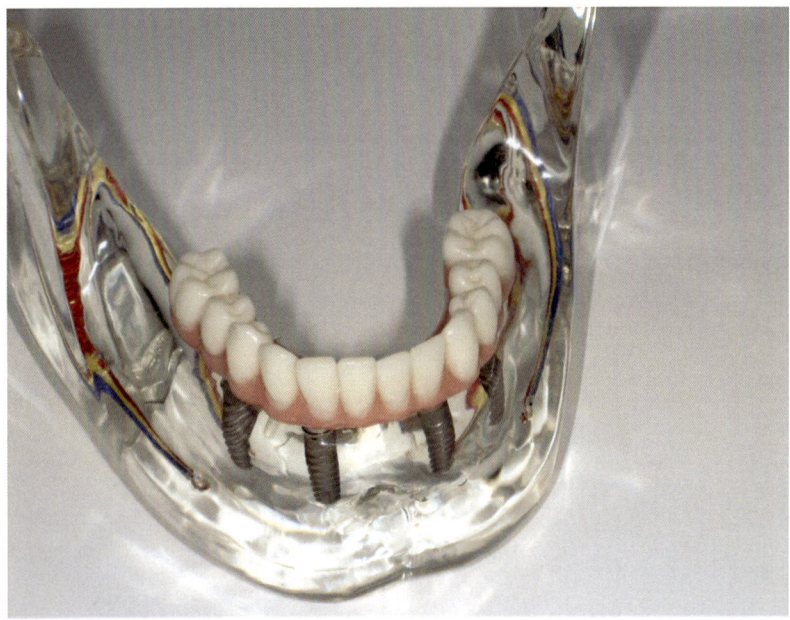

CHAPTER 05

ALL ON X: EVERYTHING BEFORE SURGERY

The Ideal Candidate

I will give a list of the ideal candidate for me

1. No health history or diseases
2. No medications
3. No Drug Allergies
4. Non smoker
5. Ideal Vitals
6. Non-Anxious patient whatsoever
7. High Pain tolerance
8. Large dense volumes of usable bone
9. Non gummy smile
10. Very kind and motivated patient
11. Large checkbook

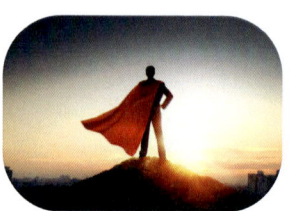

Unfortunately, such people are rare

Health histories

The American Anesthesiology Association lists operability levels in the form of the ASA chart.

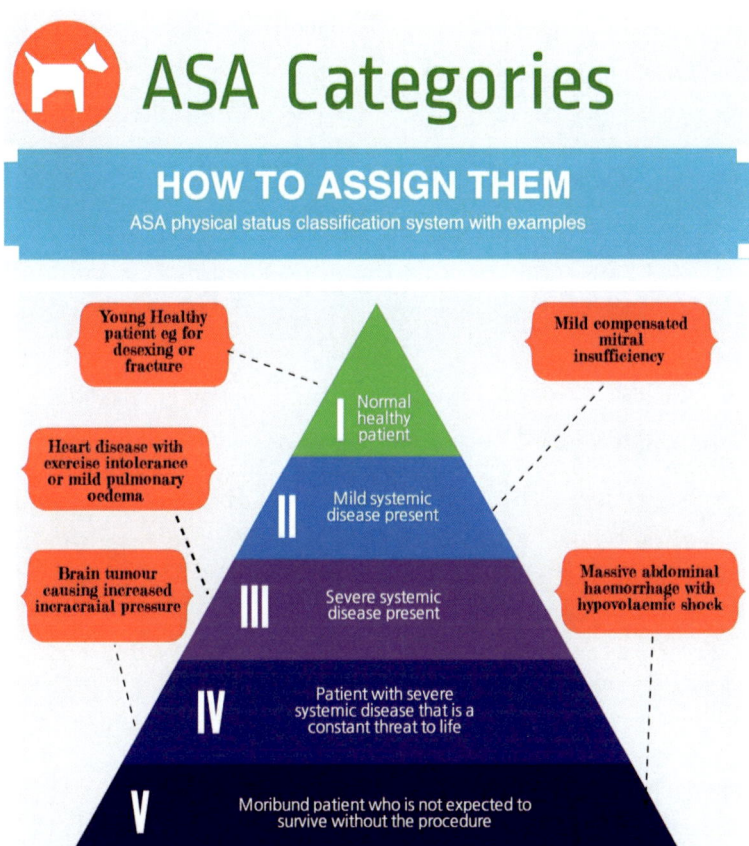

ASA?

The most important priority in any surgical procedure, including dental treatments, is the patient's safety and well-being. To mitigate risks during surgery, certain health conditions and factors must be carefully considered and, if possible, managed or stabilized before proceeding. Key risk factors that necessitate particular caution include:

- A heart attack experienced within the past year
- A stroke occurring within the past year
- Recent chemotherapy or radiation therapy for cancer
- Uncontrolled diabetes
- Bone diseases treated with intravenous bisphosphonates

In situations where there's any level of uncertainty about a patient's health status or risk factors, obtaining a medical consultation is advisable.

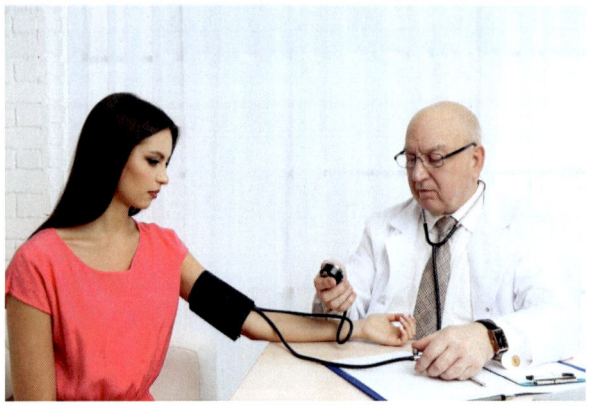

Drug allergies

Maintaining a comprehensive list of any potential allergies is crucial, especially in the context of dental implant procedures. A notable challenge arises for patients with allergies to Penicillin or Amoxicillin. For those allergic to Amoxicillin, Clindamycin has traditionally been the alternative antibiotic. However, recent data suggests Clindamycin may contribute to an increased risk of implant failure. Given this concern, it is highly recommended for individuals who suspect they have an Amoxicillin allergy to undergo conf-irmation testing with an allergist before proceeding with surgery, minimizing potential complications.

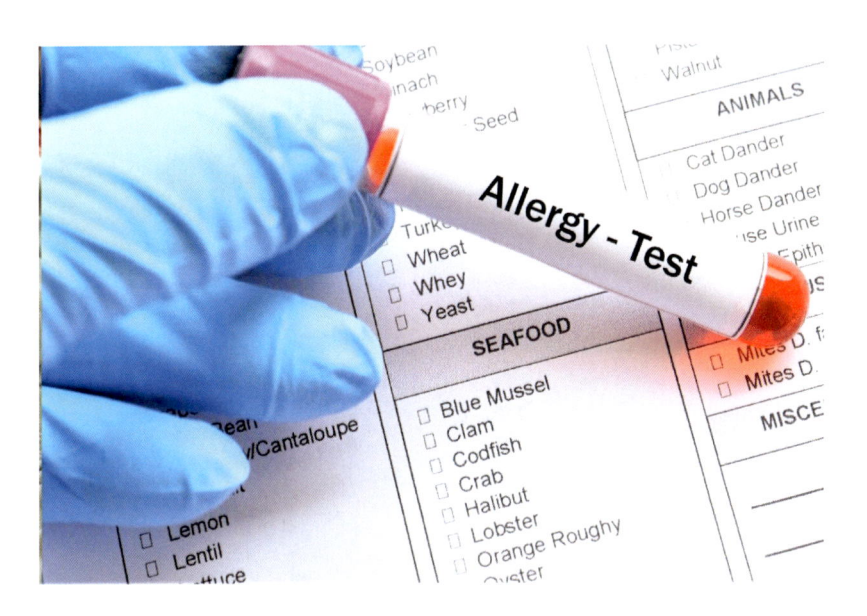

Smoking

Smoking significantly increases the risk of complications with dental implants, potentially reducing their long-term success rate to approximately 70-80%. The adverse effects of smoking on healing and the integration of implants into the jawbone cannot be overstated. Given the investment of time, effort, and resources into the implant surgery, introducing any factor that might compromise its success is ill-advised. It is strongly recommended to cease smoking at least two weeks prior to the surgery and to abstain for as long as possible afterward. Some dentists can prescribe smoking cessation medicine. This approach not only enhances the chances of successful implant integration but also contributes to overall better healing and oral health.

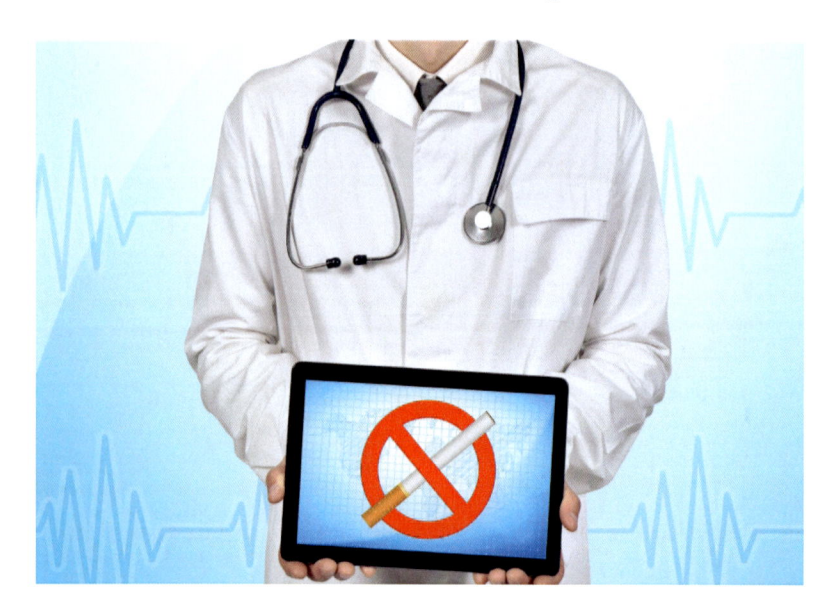

Ideal Vitals

Regardless of a patient's medical history, it is essential to record their vital signs before surgery to ensure there are no alarming indicators. Ensuring nothing appears suspicious in a patient's vital statistics is a critical step in pre-surgical preparation. Moreover, it is highly beneficial for all parties involved—patients, surgeons, and medical staff alike—to obtain a health clearance prior to surgery. This clearance acts as a precautionary measure, verifying that the patient is in a suitable condition to undergo the procedure safely. Such diligence helps in minimizing risks and optimizing outcomes for surgical interventions.

NORMAL VITAL SIGNS IN ADULTS

CORE TEMPERATURE	98.6°F (37°C)
HEART RATE	60–100 beats per minute
RESPIRATORY RATE	12–18 breaths per minute
BLOOD OXYGEN	95–100%
BLOOD PRESSURE	120/80 mm Hg

Anxiety:

Feeling anxious about visiting a doctor's office is a common experience, particularly when facing surgical procedures. To alleviate this anxiety, many dental offices are equipped to offer various forms of sedation, including nitrous oxide (commonly known as laughing gas), or a combination of sedation methods. For those whose health status allows, mild or oral sedation is often available to help patients relax before undergoing surgery.

For those requiring or preferring deeper levels of relaxation, complete or moderate sedation/anesthesia options are also available. However, it's important to note that opting for these more intensive sedation methods can increase the overall cost of the surgery.

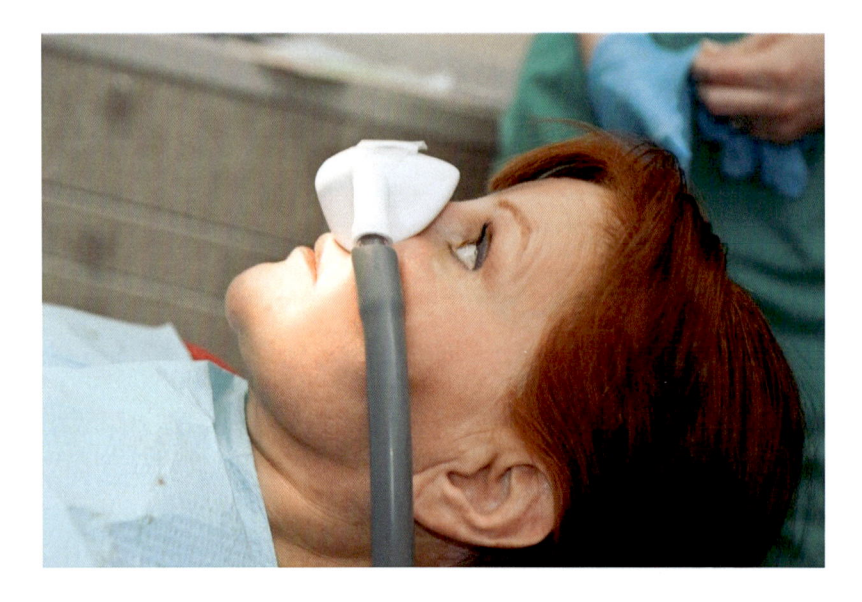

Bone Levels

Optimal bone quality is essential for implant placement. The primary function of jawbone is to support teeth. However, in the absence of teeth for an extended period, the jawbone may deteriorate, making it challenging to proceed with implants. While innovations in dental technology continue to evolve, it's crucial to utilize the current technologies effectively. In cases of insufficient upper jawbone, some surgeons have the expertise to place Pterygoid and Zygomatic implants. These implants leverage bone from other areas of the skull, offering a viable solution for patients lacking adequate bone structure.

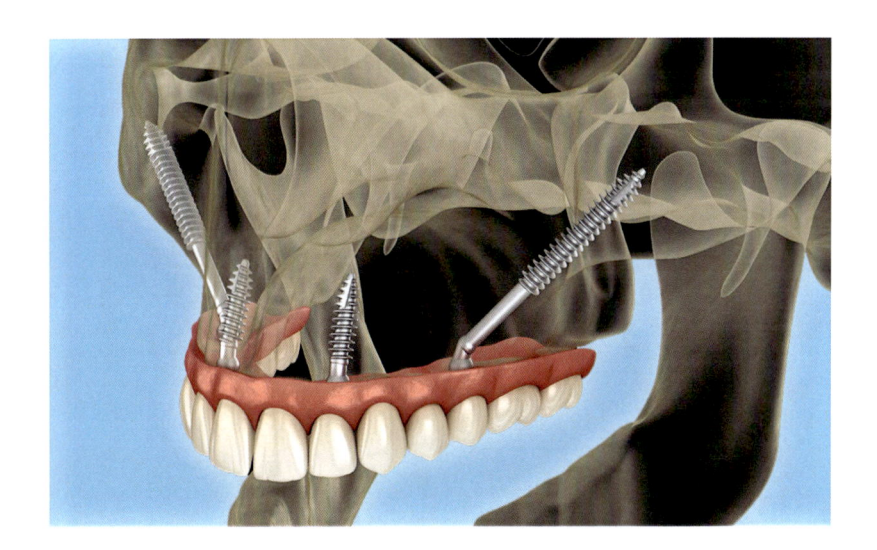

Gummy smiles

A common issue with these implants is the visible transition between the gums and the teeth. Although this transition is inevitable, ideally, it should be concealed by the lips. However, patients with particularly gummy smiles may encounter challenges in achieving this concealment. In such cases, the surgical team might need to consider surgical augmentation of the bones or tissues to make the transition between the artificial teeth and natural gums hidden under the lips. Sometimes this may be the most challenging step in the surgical outcome, if the individual's patient's anatomy presents challenges, including limited bone above the lip line.

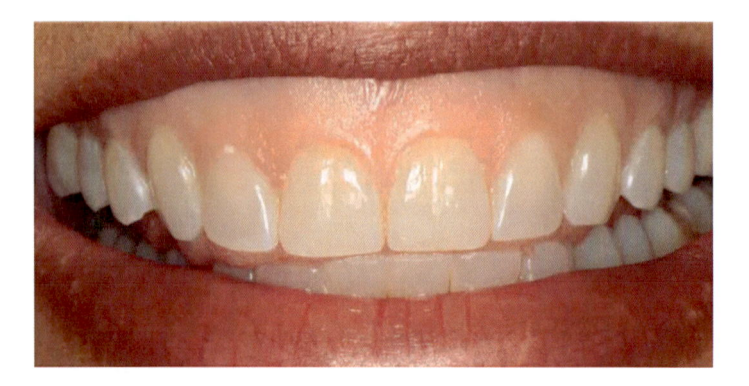

Patient-Doctor interactions

"A crucial element of the procedure is the rapport between the doctor and the patient. This relationship, often long-term, is founded on mutual appreciation and respect. Should either party sense a negative dynamic that might complicate the procedure, it's imperative that this be acknowledged and addressed prior to surgery. Ensuring a positive and cooperative relationship is essential for the success of the treatment.

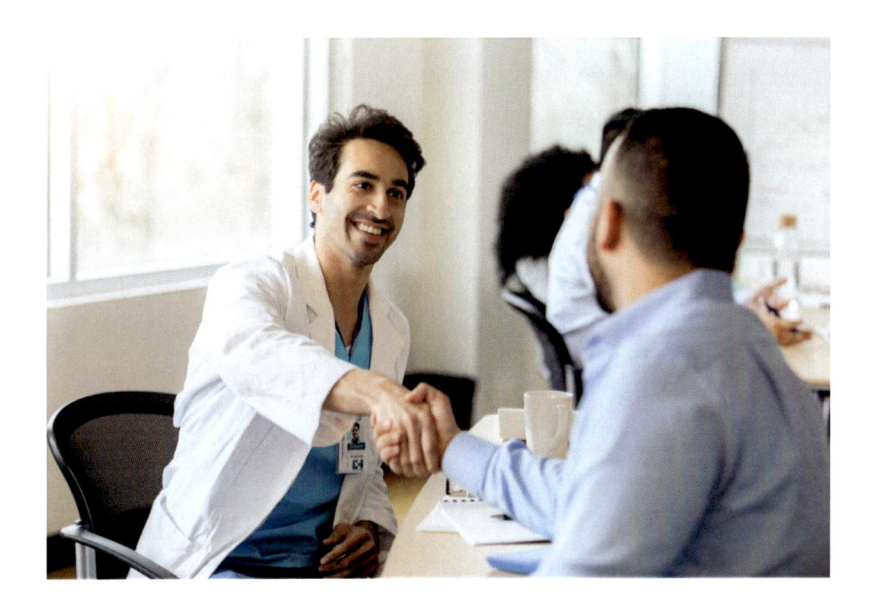

Price

The primary barrier to more widespread adoption of these dental procedures is the cost. Comprehensive treatments for the entire mouth can range between $30,000 and $100,000 USD. Dental insurance often falls short of covering these expenses, leading many to pay out of pocket. Typically, patients resort to loans with steep interest rates and stringent credit requirements. However, there are exceptions where certain medical insurance plans may cover these procedures, though these are rare and come with rigorous eligibility criteria. It's advisable to discuss with your healthcare provider about available payment options and explore any potential insurance coverage.

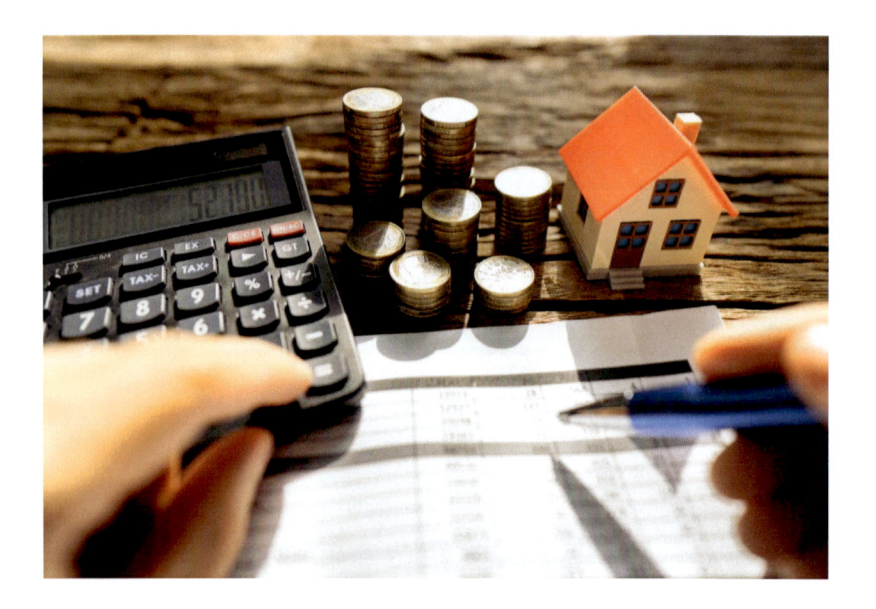

Ideal Patient:

Not everyone is the ideal candidate for dental procedures, and that's perfectly fine. A highly skilled dental team is equipped to address any challenges that arise, ensuring an outstanding outcome for all involved. The key to success is open and thorough communication with your dentist. Be proactive in sharing all relevant information and concerns—avoiding surprises on the day of surgery. Most obstacles can be navigated successfully with proper planning. As we approach the surgery, remember: effective communication is paramount. COMMUNICATION IS KEY!

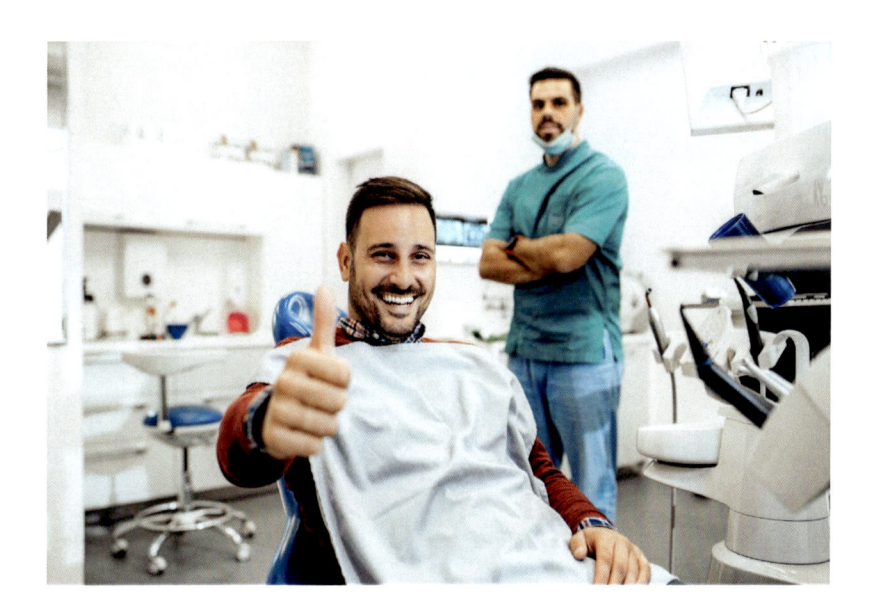

CHAPTER 06

SURGERY DAY

The night before:

Take your medications except for aspirin, blood thinners, or certain herbal supplements. Ensure you review all your medications with your doctor to discuss which ones you should continue taking and which to avoid. It's important to eat a balanced dinner without overindulging. Avoid alcohol and recreational drugs, especially before surgery, as they can interact with sedation medications. Some dentists may prescribe Valium to help you sleep well the night before. Ensure you get a good night's sleep!

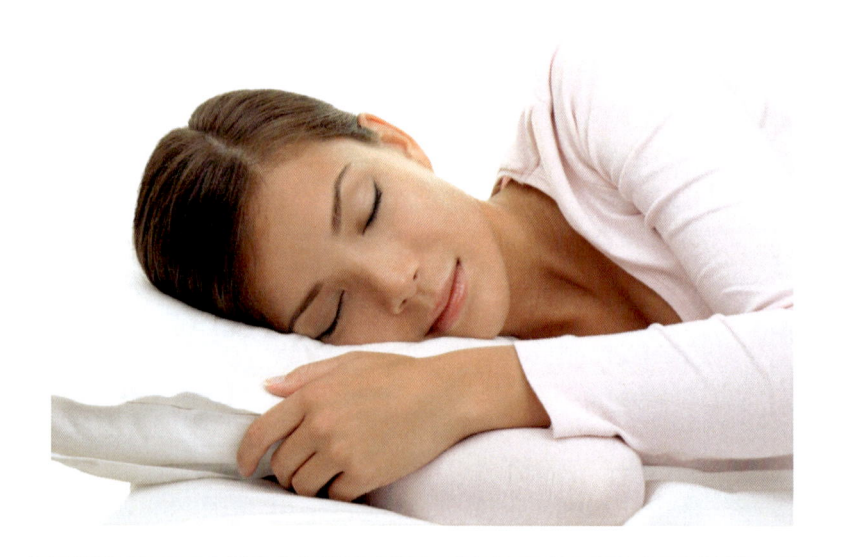

Surgery Day   44

The morning of:

Your doctor may recommend taking certain medications beforehand. It's important to discuss this with your medical team, but ensure you continue taking your regular daily medications. You may also be advised to refrain from eating or drinking before surgery to prevent nausea or vomiting. Approach the day with a positive attitude—this is a pivotal moment where your life changes!

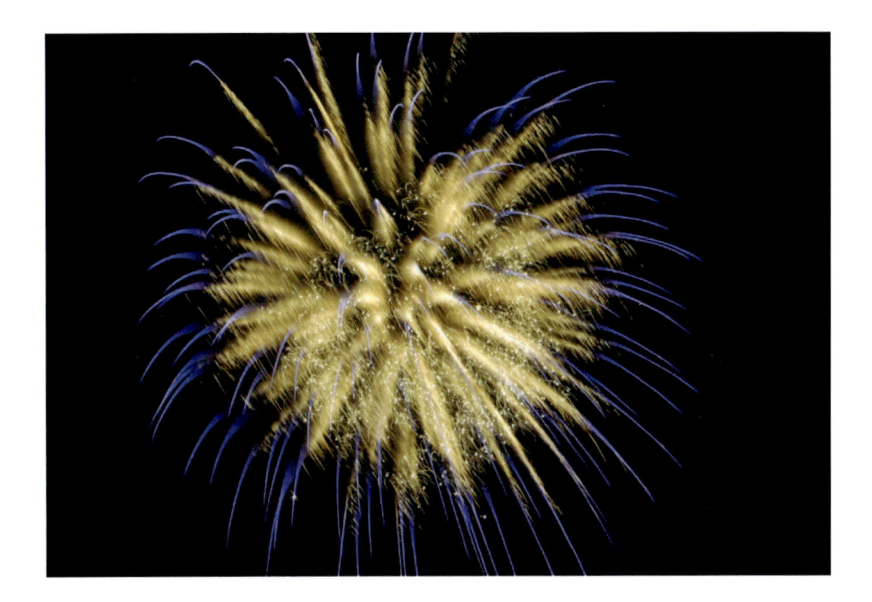

Surgery Time:

Making this chapter was difficult. The key question was how much detail and information should I include to ensure it is sufficiently informative without causing undue alarm, particularly for patients prone to high anxiety. Ideally, a patient with prior dental procedure experience would be familiar with various numbing techniques that dentists have employed for decades. At the most fundamental level, surgeons typically utilize anesthetics such as Lidocaine or Articaine. It's important to note that, even under sedation, patients will still require injections.

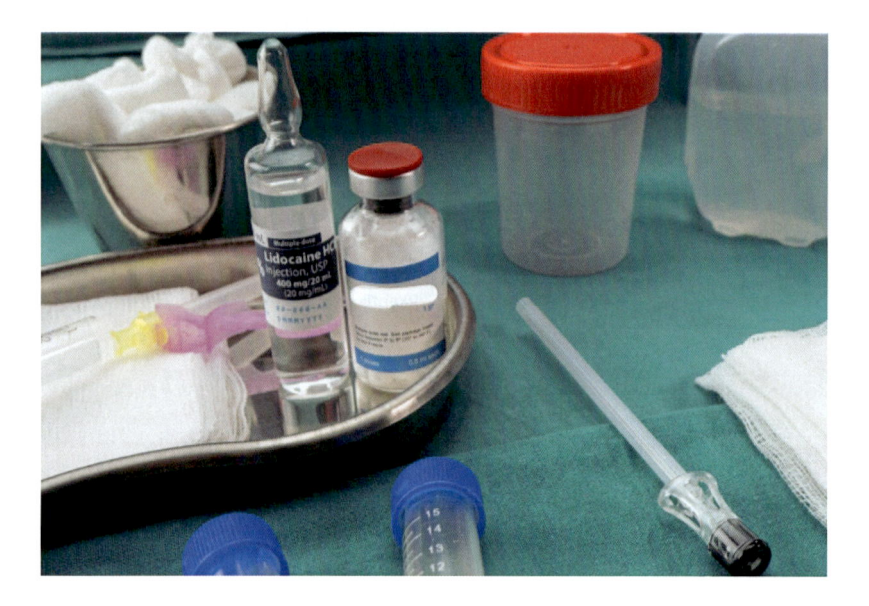

Sedation

A frequently asked question is whether one will remain awake during the procedure. I have undergone surgeries both with and without sedation, and personally, I find sedation preferable. Sedation allows you to respond to stimuli, offering a middle ground as illustrated in the chart below, which ranges from no sedation to general anesthesia. While general anesthesia is an option for these surgeries, it's important to note that employing an anesthesiologist can be quite expensive, costing approximately $1,000 per hour. However, this may be a viable option for some patients. Should you opt for this route, the surgical team will provide you with all necessary instructions.

Description	MINIMAL SEDATION	MODERATE SEDATION	DEEP SEDATION	GENERAL ANESTHESIA
Responsiveness	Normal Response To Verbal Stimulation	Interrupted Response To Verbal Stimulation	Interrupted Response To Verbal Stimulation	No Response
Airway	Unaffected	Unaffected	Intervention may be needed	Intervention needed
Ventilation	Unaffected	Unaffected	Intervention may be needed	Intervention needed
Delivery Method	Nitrous oxide gas	Oral Pills	IV	IV and Gas
Staff	Constant monitoring	Constant monitoring	Constant monitoring, advanced staff	Anesthesiologist

Digital Markers:

Explaining the digital process involves a complex principle. It's essential to establish a reference point for your mouth both before and after surgery, given that the procedure significantly alters various aspects, such as the removal of teeth and the size of the jaws. Despite these changes, it remains crucial for computers to replicate existing bite and teeth relationships. Digital markers are maintained before and after surgery to ensure an accurate overlay of the mouth's condition pre- and post-operation.

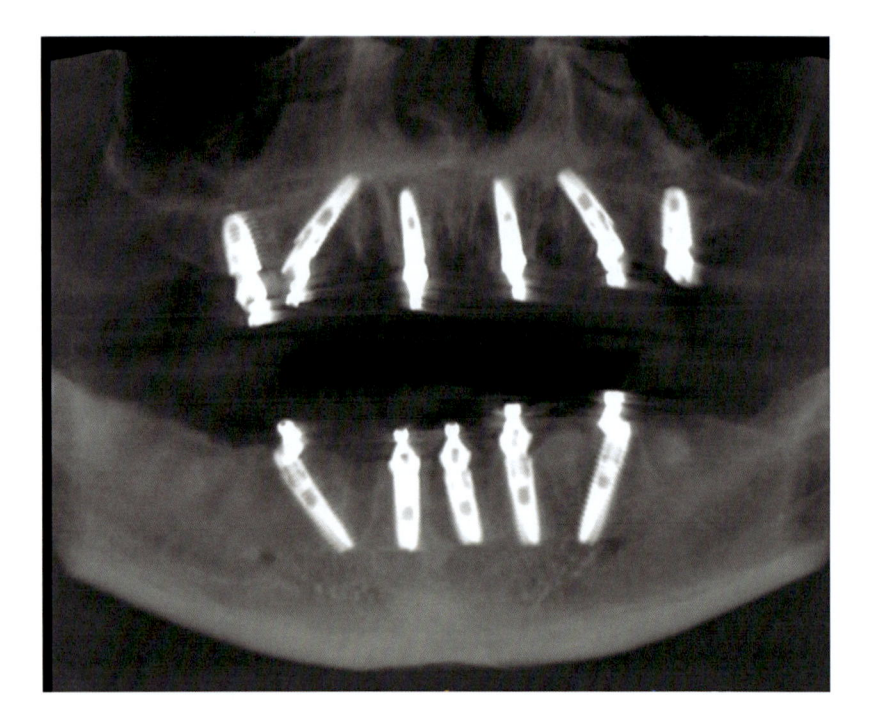

Surgery Day | 48

Pre scan:

Once the markers are positioned, the team will scan your mouth with the markers in place, using either a digital scanner or impression material. These scans are then uploaded and forwarded to the laboratory as a baseline reference. I will attach both the pre-operative and post-operative scans so you can observe how the markers align for accurate positioning.

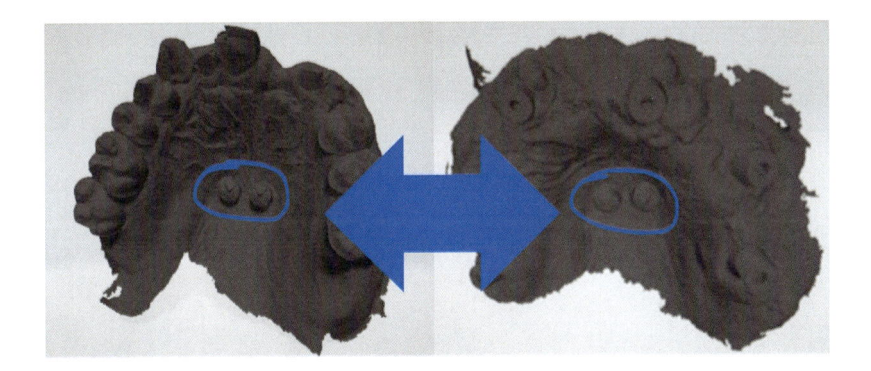

Remove teeth and bone reduction:

This section is where I'll be most sparing with the details. You're encouraged to research further on your own, but essentially, any remaining teeth need to be extracted. The bone must be shaped to ensure the final teeth have sufficient thickness. Insufficient bone reduction may result in brittle teeth prone to breaking, whereas excessive bone removal can weaken the jaw or leave inadequate space for the implants. Achieving this delicate balance is a responsibility entrusted to your surgical team.

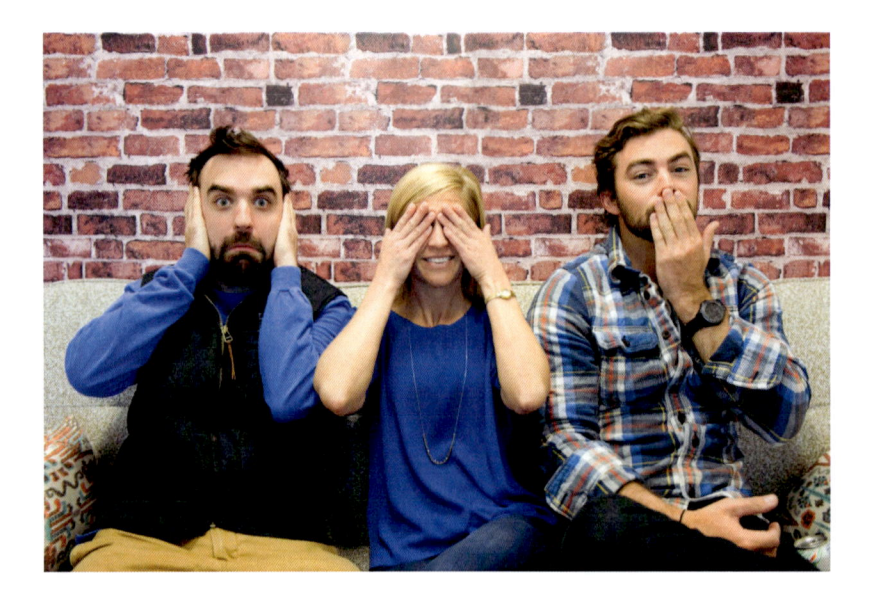

Surgery Day | 50

Placing Implants:

The decision ultimately rests with your surgical team. A minimum of four implants is required to support the teeth, though I prefer to place a few additional ones for extra stability. It's important to note that the bone in the upper jaw is generally weaker than in the lower jaw, meaning that sometimes four implants may not provide sufficient support in the upper region. However, I am not suggesting that four implants are inadequate; in some cases, that might be the maximum number a particular individual can accommodate.

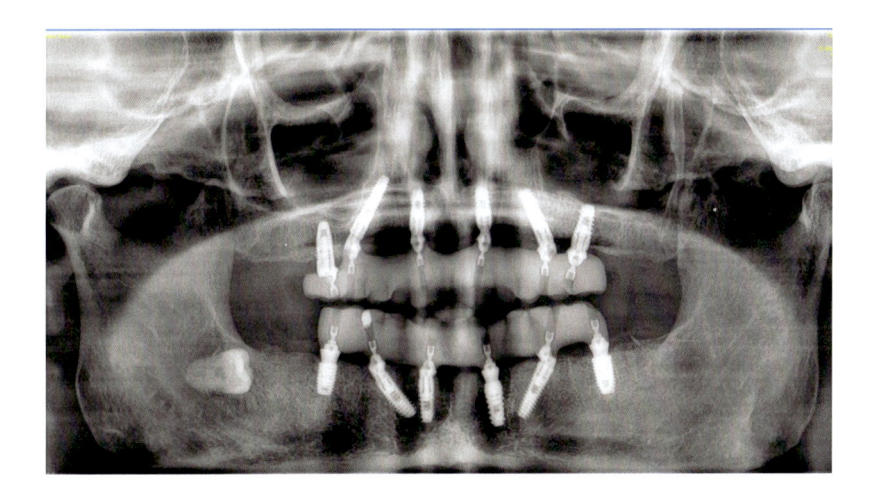

Post scans

After the implants are placed, a laboratory technician will need to digitally scan the implants using a technique known as photogrammetry. This technology may not be available in all dental offices, as it is a relatively new development in dentistry that did not become widely used until around 2020. Accessibility to such technologies might vary by region or country. However, photogrammetry significantly simplifies the process. Here is what the scan typically look like.

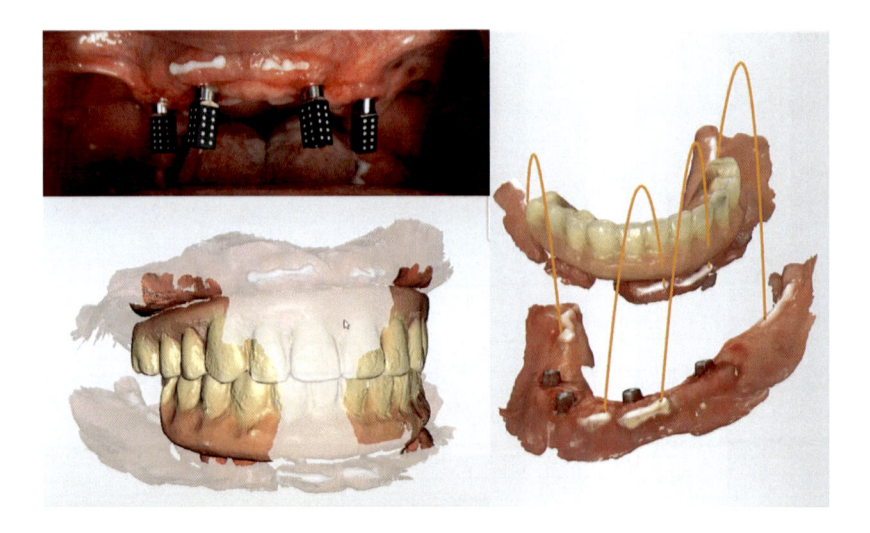

Conversions:

Many dental offices continue to employ analog methods for converting dentures, one advantage of which is receiving your completed dentures the same day. Personally, I am relieved to no longer engage in these procedures, as I found them to be labor-intensive and highly sensitive to technique, particularly post-surgery. In this traditional approach, a conventional denture is modified to accommodate implants. However, I consider the new digital methods to be significantly superior, though traditional techniques also have their merits and should not be dismissed outright.

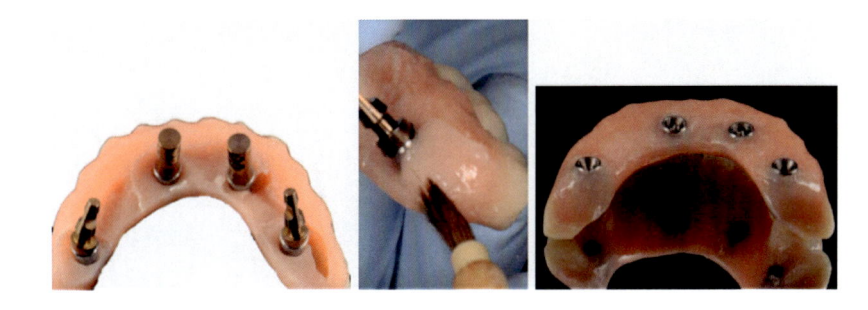

Closing up and finishing surgery:

Once the procedure is completed, the patient is ready to return home. The scans are sent to a digital designer at the laboratory, where the digital design is created. Subsequently, the teeth are 3D printed and customized for each individual patient. While some clinics may wait a day or two before fitting the final teeth, delaying excessively can result in significant swelling, potentially causing the newly made teeth to no longer fit properly.

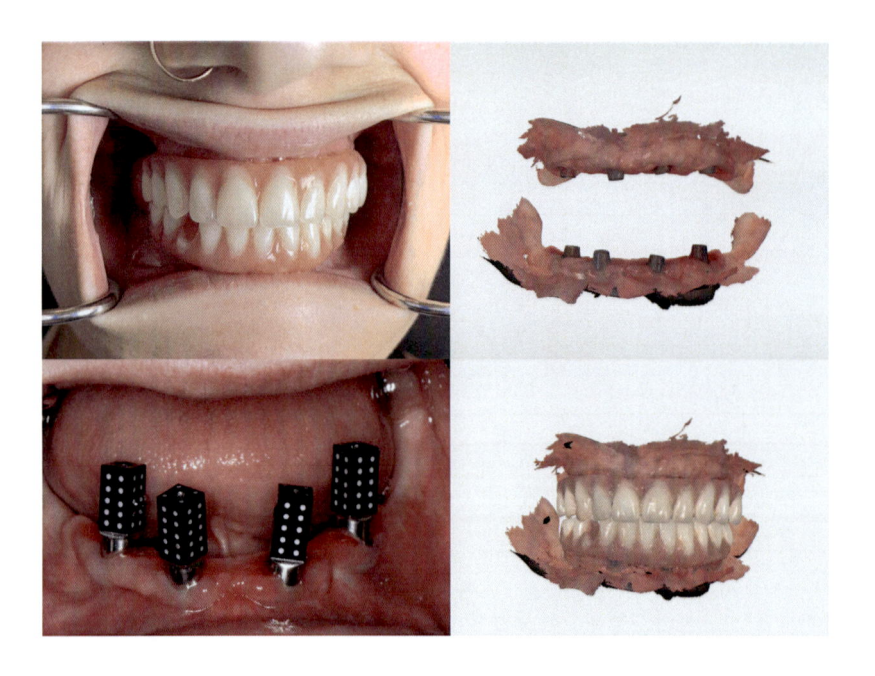

Tap, Tap, Tap:

Ensuring an accurate bite is crucial. The teeth should make even contact on all sides. Excessive force or pressure on one side can overload the implants, leading to potential failure. It is important to confirm with your dentist that all teeth are touching evenly. Thanks to 3D printing technology, adjustments to dentures can be made swiftly. There are specific contact points that may not be immediately apparent to patients, highlighting the importance of a skilled dental team capable of identifying and correcting these nuances.

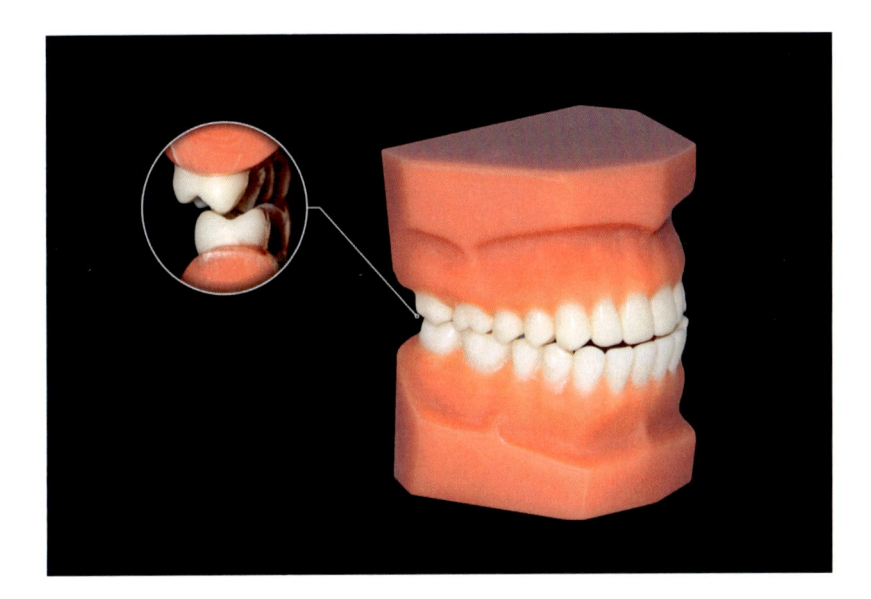

Pain meds:

After surgery, it is essential to prescribe appropriate antibiotics, anti-inflammatory medications, and pain relievers. The aim is not to foster dependency; thus, prescribing potent painkillers should be limited to avoid long-term adverse effects on the patient, ensuring only enough medication for a few days. Should excessive pain persist beyond this period, it should be managed with less addictive medications. I administer an anti-inflammatory injection to my patients post-operatively, which generally aids in managing severe pain effectively.

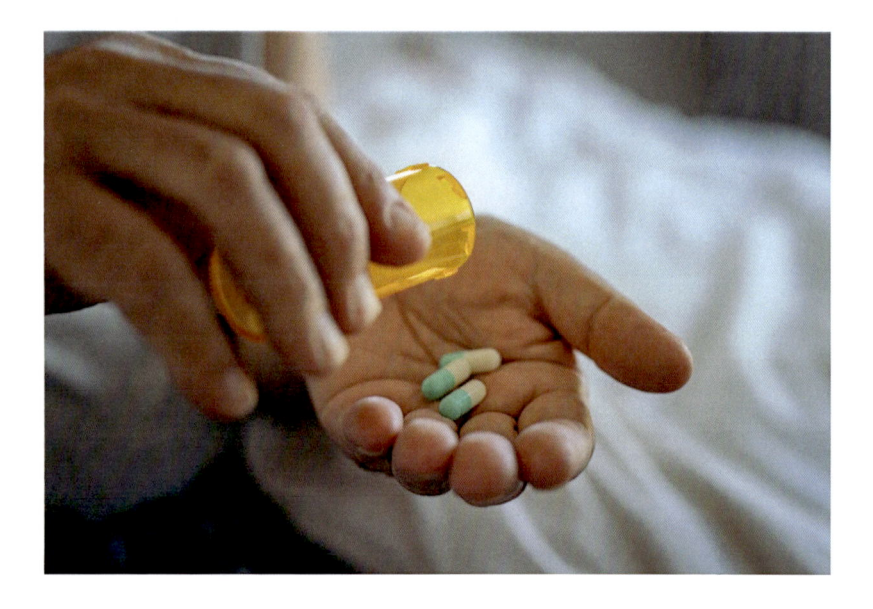

CHAPTER 07

AFTER SURGERY AND BEYOND

What Should I eat?

As we spoke earlier the implants will need time to integrate. Until they do you need to be on a soft diet. Probably a liquid diet for a day or 2 after surgery would be ideal to. What is a soft diet?

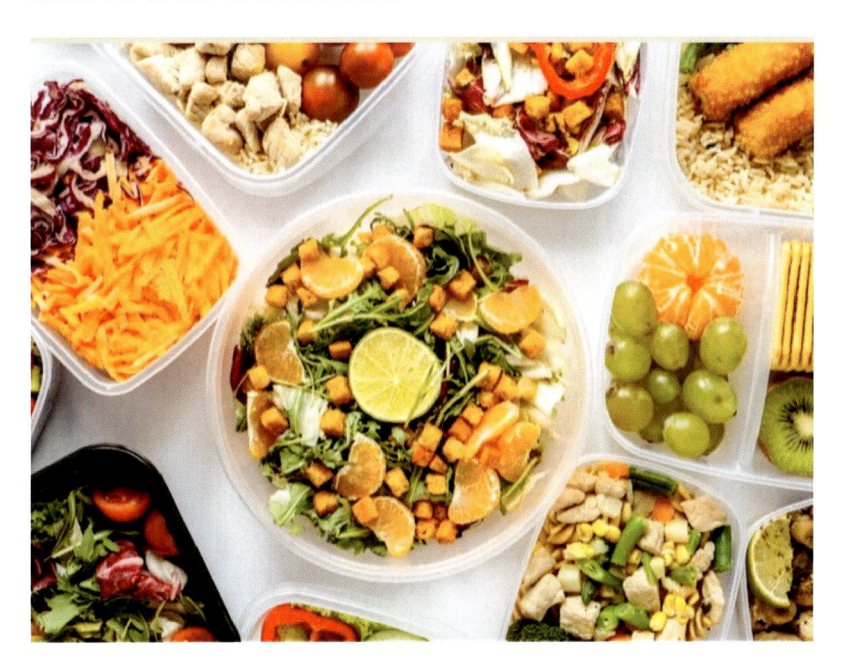

Soft Diet Chart:

A large number of foods qualify as soft foods:

- Mush or porridge-type hot cereals like oatmeal, grits and Cream-of-Wheat
- Cereals that soften easily in milk like Rice Krispies and Corn Flakes
- Soft breads and muffins
- Pasta cooked to a soft consistency
- Potatoes and sweet potatoes without skin
- Soft fruits like ripe bananas and melon
- Pureed berries put through a strainer to remove skins and seeds
- Cooked fruits without seeds or skins like apples and pears
- Fruit juice
- Avocados
- Vegetable juice

Soft Diet Chart 2:

- Skinless vegetables that cook to a soft consistency or can be mashed, like carrots, cauliflower
- Soft fish carefully de-boned
- Canned tuna or chicken
- Scrambled or soft-boiled eggs
- Tender meats and ground meats that have been well-cooked - braised meats or meats cooked in a crock-pot are especially good for this purpose
- Tofu
- Well-cooked legumes with soft skins like baked beans
- Pureed or blended soups
- Pureed or blended sauces
- Yogurt
- Cottage cheese or ricotta cheese
- Finely grated/melted cheese
- Ice cream
- Pudding or custard
- Protein powders

Foods to avoid:

- Chewy breads, especially those with whole seeds or grains and raisins
- Bagels
- English muffins
- Crusty breads such as sourdough
- Chips and crisps
- Popcorn
- Corn and peas
- Legumes with noticeable tough skins - like black beans or kidney beans
- Hard cereals
- Rice
- Raw vegetables and cooked vegetables that can't be easily mashed
- Dried fruits
- Fruits with seeds
- Pineapple
- Raw apples
- Fruit skin
- Tough meats or stringy meats
- Meat products in a casing like hot dogs and bratwurst
- Meats that take some chewing, like chicken breasts and steak
- Sliced or cubed cheese

Temporary Teeth

Concentrating solely on the digitally fabricated temporary teeth, these are constructed from polymethyl methacrylate, or PMMA for short. PMMA is a durable, strong plastic designed to endure significant chewing forces. However, it is still susceptible to breaking if subjected to sufficient force in vulnerable areas. Recent advancements in PMMA materials include reinforcement with Zirconia, which is the material intended for the final product. Theoretically, these reinforced materials could serve as final solutions, but it is likely a few years before they become a widely accepted final option.

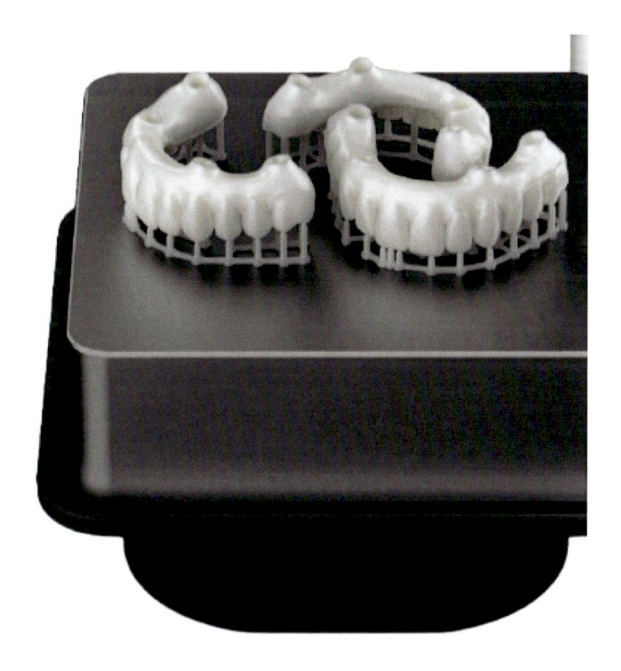

Why Temporary teeth?

Why not proceed directly to the final teeth? The challenge lies in the fact that the teeth are designed to fit immediately post-surgery. However, a few months later, as the tissue and bone levels adjust slightly, if the final teeth are placed too early, gaps can form between the gums and teeth, creating spaces where food can get trapped. Moreover, it is more effective to establish proper aesthetics, phonetics, and bite alignment with temporary teeth before finalizing the permanent ones. This approach allows for adjustments to be made in the temporary phase, ensuring a better fit and function for the final teeth.

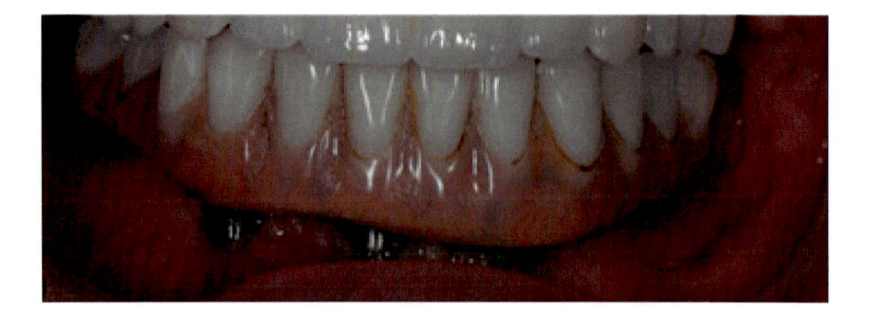

After Surgery And Beyond   62

How should I chew?

This was an aspect I hadn't contemplated until I observed variations in how some patients chew, particularly with artificial teeth. It's crucial to adopt a vertical biting motion rather than relying on the molars for a round motion. Admittedly, this concept can be challenging to convey, but your dentist should be able to provide a clearer explanation. It might not resonate with you unless you're accustomed to chewing horizontally. The basic diagram I've included aims to illustrate the difference between horizontal and vertical chewing as effectively as possible.

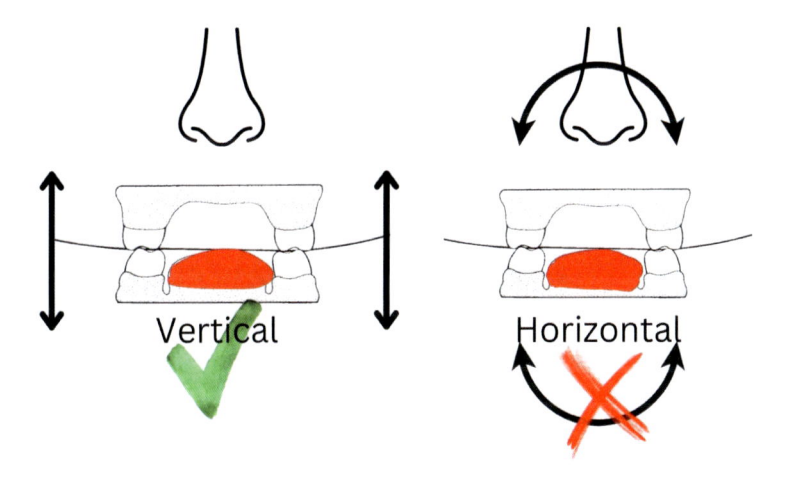

Time For finals: Which material?

When choosing materials, one must weigh the options between Full Zirconia and Acrylic fused to a titanium bar. Zirconia, while exceptionally durable, may be excessively hard, particularly when it comes into contact with natural teeth. Additionally, some individuals may find the sound produced by Zirconia on Zirconia contact during biting to be unpleasant. Despite these considerations, I personally favor Zirconia for its resilience; it tends to break less frequently and presents fewer long-term issues. This preference is informed by an experience with a patient whose acrylic/titanium dentures broke. Although we managed to repair them, the incident proved to be a hassle for everyone involved.

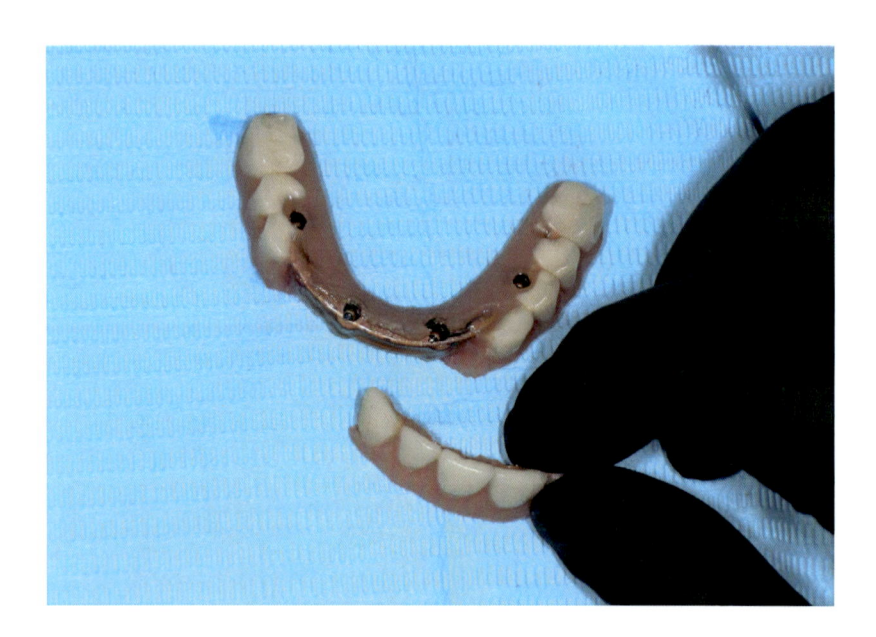

Time For finals: Scans vs impressions

Utilizing the digital method simplifies the preparation for final teeth, requiring only a few additional scans akin to those performed during surgery. This process should be quick and relatively painless. In contrast, many offices still employ traditional methods, which often necessitate 3-6 visits and numerous exchanges with the laboratory to finalize. This conventional approach can extend over several months.

The primary limitation of this method is that temporary teeth can be challenging to replace or modify. Patients may find the aesthetics of these temporary teeth unsatisfactory; they may break or chip, necessitating repairs or alterations that are significantly time-consuming, often requiring multiple appointments and interactions with a laboratory. Conversely, the 3D printing method offers a swift and efficient solution, allowing for easy reprinting that can be accomplished in as little as an hour.

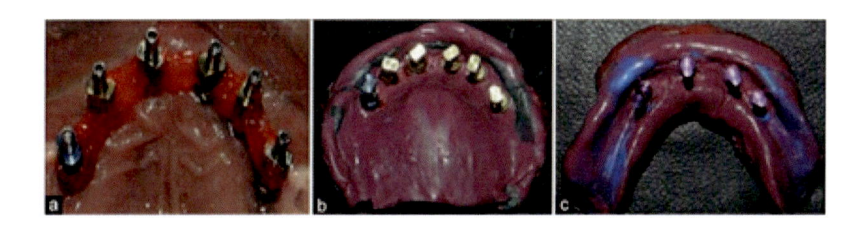

Maintenance

This step is crucial. Acquiring new teeth doesn't guarantee their permanence. We strongly advise several follow-up visits to ensure the bite is as close to perfect as possible. Additionally, the teeth require regular cleaning. My office provides a 5-year warranty, conditional on patients undergoing two cleanings per year. Our protocol involves one cleaning with the prosthesis in place and another with the prosthesis removed for a thorough cleaning and to check the screws. It's vital to avoid reverting to the habits that led to the loss of your natural teeth initially.

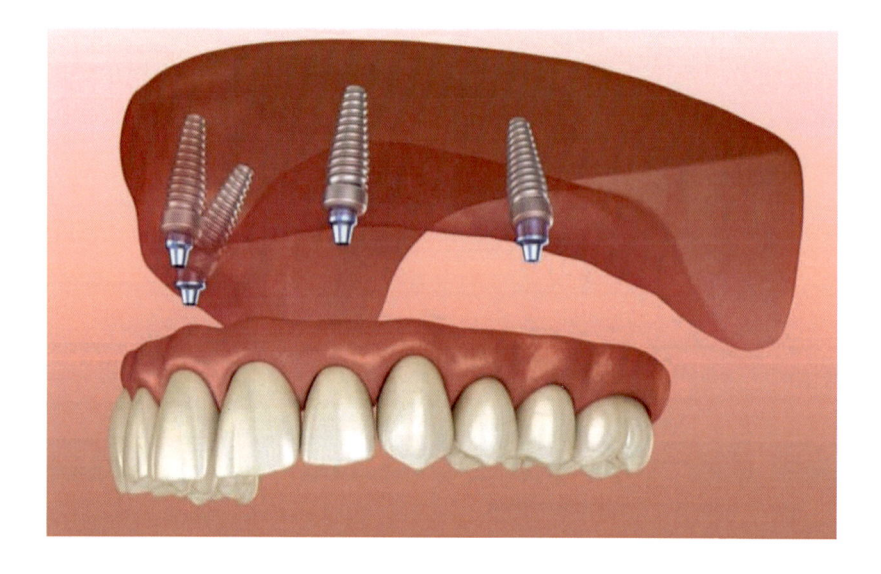

CONCLUSIONS:

Although there is much more to learn and understand about these procedures, this guide aims to provide a concise overview to aid you in making an informed decision. A question I have yet to address is the longevity of these teeth. It's difficult to predict; individuals who have lost all their teeth once are certainly at risk of experiencing it again. It's crucial to understand that this is not merely a second set of teeth but rather a second chance at maintaining oral health. Without proper care, the new teeth could fail, potentially damaging any healthy bone remaining, leaving individuals with few options. While I regret ending on a sober note after providing extensive information, emphasizing the importance of diligent care and maintenance cannot be overlooked. My goal is to equip you with sufficient knowledge to make informed and thoughtful decisions. These solutions are not inexpensive fixes to complex issues, and every step should be thoroughly considered.

ABOUT THE AUTHOR

Dr. Isaac Qureshi was born and raised in the suburbs of Chicago. He pursued his undergraduate studies at the University of Illinois at Urbana-Champaign, earned a Master of Public Health from Benedictine University, and completed his Doctorate of Dental Surgery at the University of Illinois Chicago.

Dr. Qureshi currently practices in La Grange, IL, where he has performed numerous full-mouth surgical rehabilitations. He is married and the proud father of two children.

www.HealthySmilesLaGrange.Com